JB

From Management
to Leadership

Jo Manion

From Management to Leadership

Practical Strategies for Health Care Leaders

Second Edition

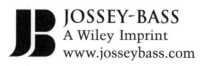

JOSSEY-BASS
A Wiley Imprint
www.josseybass.com

Published by Jossey-Bass
A Wiley Imprint
989 Market Street, San Francisco, CA 94103-1741 www.josseybass.com

The views expressed in this book are strictly those of the author and do not represent the official positions of the American Hospital Association.

 is a service mark of the American Hospital Association used under license by AHA Press.

Jossey-Bass books and products are available through most bookstores. To contact Jossey-Bass directly call our Customer Care Department within the U.S. at 800-956-7739, outside the U.S. at 317-572-3986, or fax 317-572-4002.

Jossey-Bass also publishes its books in a variety of electronic formats. Some content that appears in print may not be available in electronic books.

Library of Congress Cataloging-in-Publication Data

Manion, Jo.
From management to leadership : practical strategies for health care leaders / Jo Manion.— 2nd ed.
    p. ; cm.
    Includes bibliographical references and index.
    ISBN 0-7879-7929-5 (alk. paper)
    1. Health services administration—Psychological aspects.   2. Leadership.
3. Interpersonal relations.
    [DNLM: 1. Health Services Administration.   2. Efficiency, Organizational.   3. Health Facility Administrators.   4. Interpersonal Relations.   5. Leadership.   WX 155 M278f 2005]   I. Title.
    RA971.M3468 2005
    362.1'068—dc22   2005008651

Printed in the United States of America
SECOND EDITION
PB Printing   10 9 8 7 6 5 4 3 2 1

Contents

*This book is sincerely dedicated to all of the leaders
who have brought such richness into my life:*

*To participants in my leadership and professional programs
who have challenged, questioned, and given me countless
opportunities for new learning. It has been fun to work with you!*

*To my health care colleagues who inspire me with their sense of
commitment, courage, and perseverance in the face
of daunting challenge and obstacles. You are awesome!*

*To my family and friends for their love, support, and
encouragement. What would I do without you?*

Preface

The development of leaders remains a critical challenge facing health care organizations today. Tumultuous change is occurring at breakneck speed, creating the need for individuals who can lead others effectively during these demanding times. Required are leaders who create the direction, win the commitment of followers and other key stakeholders, and influence others to do what needs to be done to achieve a future strategic vision. Unprecedented changes are occurring in health care's executive and managerial roles and in the manner in which health care organizations function. Health care leaders must assume nontraditional roles for which they may feel inadequately equipped; new roles demand mastery of new and different skills. Present leaders face a tremendous challenge in balancing the demands of day-to-day organizational life while continually learning for the future.

Some organizations meet the challenge of leadership development by recruiting strong leaders from the outside. However, vibrant, dynamic, and flourishing organizations are also committed to developing leaders from within the existing ranks of their managers and other employees. Working in partnership with employees to develop their leadership skills is in the organization's best interests. By providing opportunities, active coaching, and guidance, the organization creates an ever-expanding source of new leaders. Without strong leaders, navigating successfully amid the turmoil of this new millennium will be difficult, if not impossible.

Leadership development is more than an organizational issue, it is an intensely personal issue for all health care workers who are being asked to assume increasingly higher levels of responsibility, to be more involved in making decisions about issues that were previously solely the traditional manager's domain, and to serve in leadership roles. Loren Ankario ("Know How to Lead," 1993) noted that in the first decade of this new millennium, "anyone who is not a leader in his or her own way probably won't have a job." More significantly, many employees are seeking—in some instances, demanding—opportunities to serve in roles that influence their work environment even more broadly. In models of shared decision making, organizations consciously develop leaders at all levels.

The concept of leaders at all levels corresponds to current societal trends. Overall, the health care workforce is more mature and experienced than ever before in our history. Today's successful health care manager understands that the old command-and-control methodology is no longer appropriate for today's workers. Instead, the work relationship has evolved into a partnership model in which leadership roles are fluid and dynamic and individuals move in and out of these roles almost constantly. Facilitating the development of employees' leadership skills makes sense because the entire organization benefits. The organization's foundation is stronger, its structure more resilient, and its future viability more likely in an organization filled with individuals who are leaders or are capable of moving into leadership roles.

This book is written for all health care leaders and aspiring leaders. Seasoned leaders will find that the concepts and skills presented here are essential as they reshape and redefine their roles. The book may also serve as a reference or reminder to which the master leader may return when faced with a particular challenge. For new or aspiring leaders, this book can serve as a road map for developing interpersonal skills that enhance the leadership process.

In his book *On Becoming a Leader*, Warren Bennis (1989) notes that leadership courses can teach only skills, not character or vision. He believes character and vision develop in an individual over time, most often as a result of life experiences—learning that occurs beyond traditional course work. However, Peter Drucker believes that all aspects of leadership can and must be learned (Hesselbein, Goldsmith, and Beckhard, 1996). Perhaps it is useful to differentiate between talent and skills, as Buckingham and Coffman (1999) suggest. First, they believe that talent combined with training, determination, and practice is what leads to excellence in practice. In other words, all the determination, education, and training in the world will not help me become a great singer if I do not first have the necessary talent to excel (that is, I am tone deaf). Furthermore, talent cannot be taught; it is there, or it is not. The presence of the right talent, more than experience, learning, or intelligence, is the prerequisite for excellence as a leader. Skills, on the other hand, can be taught and developed. The purpose of this book is to explore the essential interpersonal skills that an effective leader needs that *can* be taught and learned: skills that, with study and practice, can increase a leader's effectiveness. Only through applying and using these skills does the leader develop them.

Prior to the publication of the first edition of this book, the American Hospital Association Press and the Center for Health Care Leadership of the American Hospital Association conducted market research on the nature of the leadership gap in health care. Focus groups of more than sixty well-known chief executive officers, board members, physician leaders, consultants, academicians, and community activists revealed five administrative pitfalls driving the then-emerging paradigm of health care leadership:

Little or no sense of shared vision and mission within the health care organization

Ineffective communication skills, especially at the executive level

Unwillingness to abandon hierarchical control structures, particularly at the executive and board level

Refusal to let go of the hospital mentality and traditional modes of service

Denial of the inevitability of rapid evolution toward capitated reimbursement and managed care

Consequences of these pitfalls are significant, affecting organizational health and future viability. To offset these weaknesses, leaders need to take on some nontraditional roles for which they may feel unprepared. Mastery of new skills is critical to the successful transition into these roles, and the research shows that these nontraditional skills are clustered into two domains:

Systems thinking, including skills in collaborative envisioning, strategic planning, broad-based decision making, innovative problem solving and process improvement, and stewardship

Interpersonal abilities, including communication skills, both verbal and nonverbal; coaching; giving constructive feedback; managing conflict; building consensus; delegating responsibility, building teams, and managing change

This book addresses these interpersonal skills, although in a somewhat unusual format. The premise of this book is that leadership exists only within a relationship: if there are no followers, there is no need for a leader. Interpersonal skills in leadership are critical success factors, yet few have written about developing these skills within the leadership context. This book identifies the fundamental interpersonal competencies every leader needs, and it maps out suggestions for improving these skills. It shares examples from health care leaders at all levels to emphasize key points. The concepts in this book are immediately applicable in leadership practice at any level and in any setting where leadership is required and exists.

This second edition contains significantly updated and expanded content. The author has added current and timely references that reflect current leadership writings. The first chapter sets the stage by exploring the difference between management and leadership, a concept that even experienced managers and leaders often have trouble grasping concretely. It provides a working definition of leadership and identifies key interpersonal requirements. The chapter examines the reasons that leadership is more crucial today, as well as the challenges that the contemporary leader faces. Each of the remaining chapters fully examines a key leadership competency.

Chapter Two focuses on establishing the leader-follower relationship. It addresses the three key elements of this relationship—trust, respect, and communication—and includes the nature of collaboration and aspects of forming a partnership. Contemporary leaders will be successful only if they are willing and able to work effectively in partnership with others.

Building commitment among followers is the theme of Chapter Three. The author has significantly expanded this chapter's content; it includes extensive discussion of the concept of organizational commitment. Executives and managers who inform employees of decisions they have made are seeking compliance or conformance. Most organizational changes occurring today require full commitment from followers to be successful. Commitment is often described as *buy-in*, a feeling of ownership that goes well beyond mere compliance. Commitment engages the heart and emotions, not just the intellect. What can a leader do to increase the likelihood that key stakeholders—employees, physicians, community members—will commit to the direction the organization takes? The chapter examines both affective and normative organizational commitment. Building a sense of connection and community among all participants as well as clarifying shared values and a common purpose leads to the possibility of a shared vision that is energizing and inspiring.

Chapter Four deals with the leader's role in communicating strategically and clearly. Although seemingly the simplest of the interpersonal competencies, communication is central to establishing a healthy leader-follower relationship. This chapter thoroughly explores verbal and nonverbal communication within the context of contemporary leadership practice. It reexamines long-known principles and concepts in light of today's workplace and challenges. It addresses special communication issues such as communicating during times of rapid change, over geographical distances, and with teams. The chapter identifies barriers to effective communication, such as gender and style differences, as well as the use of "tribal" language.

Many leaders and managers learned their skills in work environments that emphasized outcomes rather than processes. Such organizations often rewarded and promoted the decisive get-it-done individual, whereas they may have seen as slow and plodding the individual who spent the time needed to ensure that the organization followed an appropriate process. Today's leaders must be able to integrate these two approaches and achieve effective outcomes through constructive processes. Key principles of facilitating process are the focus of Chapter Five. The chapter scrutinizes critical processes—such as empowering others, resolving conflict, creating effective teams, and leading change and transition. The author has separated the critical processes of problem solving and decision making from this chapter and made them the basis of a new chapter focused on getting results. An extension of Chapter Five, the new Chapter Six now includes two alternatives to a traditional problem-solving approach, the action research methodology of appreciative inquiry, and a discussion on recognizing polarities and managing them.

The major interpersonal competency, developing others, is the subject of Chapter Seven. Everyone agrees that leaders today must be coaches, but to date little practical, concrete advice is available on how to fill this role. Principles of coaching, teaching, motivating, and encouraging others are this chapter's subject. Effective leaders are continual learners themselves; and they expect others around them to continually grow, develop, learn, and stretch. Good leaders are serious about tapping the potential within each person to expand his or her reach, to grow, and to establish leadership skills. Systems thinking and collaborative learning are key characteristics of a leader-coach-teacher.

Although mastery of these key competencies does not guarantee immediately successful leadership, it can help the individual who has innate talents become more effective. Developing and refining our leadership skills is a lifelong journey. Circumstances continually alter, creating the need for new skills sets. The author offers this book to stimulate thought and to provoke creative action for those on the path to developing leadership.

Acknowledgments

The author gratefully acknowledges the following people who were instrumental in helping make this book a reality:

The countless leader-colleagues who over the years have shared their experiences and stories with me while on their path

The colleagues and research participants who willingly and generously gave of their time and energy in my pursuit of answers

Winnie Schmeling, friend and colleague, who started the ball rolling; and Richard Hill, *Hospitals & Health Networks* online editor, who worked patiently with me to make the first edition a reality

Andy Pasternack, senior editor at Jossey-Bass, whose gentle prodding and persistence for a second edition finally paid off

And finally, my husband, Craig, who once again provided essential support, love, and encouragement, as well as the space for my writing!

The Author

Jo Manion is the president of Manion & Associates, an organizational development consulting practice located in Oviedo, Florida. A nationally recognized professional speaker, consultant, and author, she specializes in practical strategies for professional and organizational development. Her almost forty years of health care experience in a variety of organizations and positions has created expertise in the areas of leadership development, the creation of positive work environments, and the development of effective teams. Her research focuses on the area of the leadership role in creating positive workplaces. A fellow in the American Academy of Nursing, she holds both a master's degree and a doctorate in the area of human and organizational systems from the Fielding Graduate Institute. She is the author of *Change From Within: Nurse Intrapreneurs as Health Care Innovators* (1990) and coauthor of *Team-Based Health Care Organizations* (1996) and *Nature's Wisdom in the Work Place: Managing Energy in Today's Health Care Organization* (2005). Additionally, *Create a Positive Health Care Workplace! Practical Strategies to Retain Today's Workforce and Find Tomorrow's* is scheduled for release in mid 2005. She is also widely published in many health care journals. Visit her Web site at www.jomanion.com.

From Management
to Leadership

1

Leadership

An Elusive Concept

*Leadership has to take place every day.
It cannot be the responsibility of the few, a rare event,
or a once-in-a-lifetime opportunity.*
R. A. Heifetz and D. L. Laurie,
"The Work of Leadership"

No issue is as important in health care today as the development
and continual evolution of leaders. "Leadership is the pivotal
force behind successful organizations. . . . To create vital and viable
organizations, leadership is necessary to help organizations develop
a new vision of what they can be, then mobilize the organization to
change toward the new vision" (Bennis and Nanus, 1985, p. 12). An
organization's success is directly correlated to its leaders' strengths.
The failure of an organization to develop leaders at all levels, relying instead on a few strong leaders at the top, results in dismal outcomes. In the foreword of Gifford and Elizabeth Pinchot's book *The
Intelligent Organization* (1996b, p. x), Warren Bennis notes that "traditional bureaucratic organizations have failed and continue to fail,
in large part, because they tend to rely exclusively on the intelligence
of those at the very top of the pyramid."

In the same way, relying only on formal managers for leadership
limits the tremendous possibilities that exist when leaders are differ-
entiated from managers. "Solutions . . . reside not in the executive

suite but in the collective intelligence of employees at all levels, who need to use one another as resources, often across boundaries, and learn their way to those solutions" (Heifetz and Laurie, 1997, p. 124). Health care is facing a daunting challenge: the development of leaders and viable succession planning. After the 1990s "the leadership pool in health care is shrinking in part because companies continue to ruthlessly excise management positions—formerly training grounds for aspiring executives—in the race to become leaner and meaner" (Grossman, 1999, p. 18). And although these tactics may save money in the short term, the long-term costs to health care are significant in the absence of qualified individuals to move into executive and leadership roles.

Unfortunately, few people understand clearly the distinction between leadership and management; as a result, this narrows the field from which organizational leaders might emerge. In some instances, organizations do not recognize leaders who emerge from the ranks; they sometimes resist them and label them as troublemakers or dissatisfied employees. This chapter explores the concept of leadership, differentiates it from management, identifies reasons leadership is so critical in today's health care organizations, and illuminates the major challenges facing current health care leaders.

Defining Leadership

Defining leadership is the first step. Most authorities on the topic define *leadership* as influencing others to do what needs to be done, especially those things the leader believes need to be accomplished. Kouzes and Posner (2002, p. xvii) identify the leadership challenge as "how leaders mobilize others to want to get extraordinary things done in organizations." Max DePree (1989, p. xx) believes the art of leadership is "liberating people to do what is required of them in the most effective and humane way possible." This definition implies that leadership is not something one does to or for the follower but is instead a process of releasing the potential already present within an individual. The leader sets the stage and then steps out of the way to let others perform. True leadership enables the follower to realize his or her full potential—potential that the follower perhaps did not suspect.

Also implied in any definition is that leadership is work. It is about performance: achieving outcomes, getting needed results. Peter Drucker (1992, p. 199) says that "it has little to do with 'leadership qualities' and even less to do with 'charisma.' It is mundane, unromantic, and boring. Its essence is performance." Kouzes and Posner (2002, p. 13) reinforce this message: "Leadership is not at all about personality; it's about practice."

Leadership is mobilizing the interest, energy, and commitment of all people at all levels of the organization. It is a means to an end. "An effective leader knows that the ultimate task of leadership is to create human energies and human vision" (Drucker, 1992, p. 122). Bardwick (1996) clearly states that leadership is not intellectual or cognitive but emotional. She points out that at the emotional level, leaders create followers because they generate "confidence in people who are frightened, certainty in people who were vacillating, action where there was hesitation, strength where there was weakness, expertise where there was floundering, courage where there were cowards, optimism where there was cynicism, and a conviction that the future will be better" (p. 14).

Noted leadership scholar and author Warren Bennis, who has spent over three decades studying leaders, describes the leader as "one who manifests direction, integrity, hardiness, and courage in a consistent pattern of behavior that inspires trust, motivation, and responsibility on the part of the followers who in turn become leaders themselves" (Johnson, 1998, p. 293). Furthermore, he offers three key ingredients for successful leadership (Bennis, 1989):

- A clear vision of what needs to be accomplished

- Passion or an intense level of personal commitment

- Integrity or character

None of these are teachable by the methods often used for leadership development, such as reading or attending seminars and formal educational courses. However, all three can be learned or perfected through life's experiences. For most people, the development of leadership ability is lifelong work—a trial-and-error method of perfecting techniques and approaches, the evolution of personality and individual beliefs. Often the leader is not even aware of exactly how he or she influenced a follower. An opportunity or need to lead appeared, and the leader stepped forward to meet the challenge.

Harry Kraemer (2003, p. 18), as chairman and CEO of Baxter Healthcare, believes that the best leaders are "people who have a very delicate balance between self-confidence and humility." They are both self-confident and comfortable expressing their ideas and opinions, but they balance this expression with a healthy dose of humility and an understanding that other people may actually have better ideas and more insight on any given issue. And perhaps most telling are the results of research conducted by Jim Collins and his associates (2001), who studied extensively the difference between good companies and compared them to similar companies that had achieved greatness. Although Collins told his research team specifically not to focus on leadership at the top, the analysis revealed that leadership was a key factor for those companies with extraordinary success. The type of leadership was a shocking surprise to the researchers. They found that the characteristics of these successful leaders did not include high-profile personalities and celebrity status but just the opposite: "Self-effacing, quiet, reserved, even shy—these leaders are a paradoxical blend of personal humility and professional will. They are more like Lincoln and Socrates than Patton or Caesar" (p. 12). Their ambition is first and foremost for their organization, not for themselves.

Differentiating Management and Leadership

How does leadership differ from management? Most would agree that not all managers are good leaders and not all leaders are good managers. However, differentiating between these two concepts concisely and concretely is difficult. A common misconception is that the legitimate authority of a position, such as holding a management job or an elected position, automatically confers leadership skills on the person holding that position. Nothing is further from the truth. Leadership and management are two separate and distinct concepts, although they may exist simultaneously in the same person. In an interview (Flower, 1990), Bennis compares management and leadership on several key points. As we will see, his viewpoint greatly increases clarity about these two concepts.

Efficiency Versus Effectiveness

The first differentiating point is related to the essential focus of the individual. A manager is concerned with efficiency, getting things done right, better, and faster. Increasing productivity and streamlining current operations are important, and managers often exhort employees to work smarter, not harder. In contrast, a leader is more concerned with effectiveness, asking: Are we doing the right thing? The initial question is not "How can we do this faster?" but "Should we be doing this at all?" To answer the latter question, a key deciding factor is whether the activity in question directly supports the organization's overall purpose and mission. Is the activity in alignment with the stated values and beliefs of the organization and the people within it? Will it produce desirable outcomes?

A classic example of this difference occurred some years ago in a 480-bed midwestern medical center. As the hospital's volume increased over the years, traffic flow on the elevators became a major problem. Several process improvement teams attacked the problem at various times but came up with no lasting or truly effective solution. After years of frustration, a team assigned to this issue finally came up with a solution that involved building a new set of elevators for patients only. The intent was to move patients faster and more efficiently, a goal the medical center accomplished for several hundred thousand dollars.

A couple of years later, the organization went through a major reengineering and work-redesign effort. The first questions were the following: Why are we transporting patients all over the organization? Can we deploy any services to the patient-care unit to reduce the distance that patients travel? These are leadership questions; instead of asking how to move patients faster, the project team asked: Should they be moved at all? How can we reduce movement of patients? In fact, today new health care facilities are being built based on the concept of the universal room: the patient is admitted to a room and remains assigned to that room throughout the entire hospital stay. The level of care may change depending on the patient's needs, but the location of the patient does not.

How Versus What and Why

A second differentiating characteristic is that management is about *how*, whereas leadership is about *what* and *why*. A good manager is usually one who understands the work processes and can demonstrate and explain to an employee how to accomplish the work. Health care, which has a history of promoting people with job expertise to management and supervisory roles, clearly values these phenomena. The highly skilled practitioner becomes a manager, and overall this is the typical pattern regardless of the department or discipline in question. Health care workers tend to value job expertise in their managers and, in fact, often show disdain for the manager who cannot perform at a highly competent level the work of the employees they manage. This is understandable when we examine health care's history. Early hospitals were led and managed by individuals with a high level of technical clinical expertise (physicians and nurses). Only in recent decades have a significant number of executives and managers with nonclinical backgrounds entered health care institutions. Some clinical health care workers today still doubt that individuals with nonclinical backgrounds can possibly understand enough to be effective leaders in health care organizations.

Knowing and controlling work processes are essential components of the managerial role—and rightly so. Management's origins were in the factories of the industrial age. The workforce of the late 1800s was very different from today's workforce. Most early factory workers were newly arrived immigrants, women, and children—poorly informed, uneducated, non-English-speaking, and uninvolved employees—working for survival wages. The work was compartmentalized, broken down into small manageable pieces that one person could easily teach to these early workers. The manager was responsible for ensuring that employees did the work correctly and was often the only person who understood the entire piece of work.

In contrast, a leader focuses on what needs to be done and why. He or she spends more time explaining the general direction and purpose of the work, and then the leader gets out of the way so that the follower can do it. Someone once characterized a leader as an individual who describes what needs to be done, then says, "It's up to you to impress me with how you do it."

This implies several different points. First, the leader knows what needs to be done and can clearly articulate this to others in a way that convinces the follower(s) that it is an appropriate direction. Second, the leader has the patience to share the reasons this course has been chosen and ensures that those reasons are acceptable and valid to the follower. Finally, the leader accepts that the follower may find a new and different way to accomplish the goals. The leader is not wedded to his or her way of performing a task or carrying out a responsibility.

Multiple examples of this leadership approach appeared in the 1990s in organizations undergoing major work-redesign or restructuring initiatives. In one medical center, the CEO addressed employees before redesigning work was begun, explaining the organization's current status, the external environment, and the reasons the board of trustees and executive team believed work redesign was necessary for the organization's future viability. The reasons were clear; in most instances, the employees viewed them as important and valued them. A team of employees was then formed that was instrumental in determining how to achieve results and carry out the project. In other organizations, work redesign has failed because it was undertaken with only a hospital-oriented mentality—a controlling leader who believed there was one right way to achieve needed outcomes—rather than a systems approach. Employees may have participated, but they did not believe in or value the reasons behind the project.

Structure Versus People

In contrast, Bennis (Flower, 1990) points out that management is about systems, controls, procedures, and policies—all of which create structure—whereas leadership is about people. Managers spend much of their time dealing with organizational structure. Anyone who has successfully participated in an accreditation visit by an outside agency has a sense of the number of policies and procedures that the average health care institution generates. There is usually a policy or procedure for every aspect of organizational and professional life. Infection control monitoring, risk management reporting, and patient-complaint resolution are only a few among the multitude of control systems designed to oversee organizational processes. These systems ensure that work is progressing as expected; they are designed to alert the manager to any deviation so that it can be investigated and corrected. Extensive policies and procedures, however, can sometimes be used to substitute for employees' good judgment and initiative in decision making. Relying heavily on the use of written policies and procedures can inadvertently weaken the development of individual decision making in the organization.

Leadership is about people and relationships. Leadership only exists within the context of a relationship. If there are no followers, there is no need for leadership, just independent action. Leadership occurs when leader behavior influences someone else to act in a certain manner, and at the core of such a connection between people is trust. Chapter Two explores these concepts in depth. Leadership as a relationship may be disturbing news for managers who have limited people or interpersonal skills, for an individual who has difficulty in working with others will find it virtually impossible to become a fully effective leader. A book on policies and procedures cannot replace this key relationship. Fortunately, an aspiring leader can develop and hone people skills, but maintaining them takes more energy if they are not part of the individual's natural talent base.

Status Quo Versus Innovation

Whereas maintaining and managing the status quo are appropriate managerial behaviors (Bennis, 1989), leaders are more concerned with innovation and creating new processes for the future. This is a difficult area for many health care leaders because most health care organizations have not customarily encouraged or highly valued either creativity or innovation. The words are frequently used and appear in many mission statements, but only rarely are health care organizations flexible and fluid enough to encourage true innovation. Most are bureaucratic structures that respond to any deviation from standard practice as something to stamp out, control, or limit in some manner.

Punitive responses to mistakes are common, and many managers have learned not to rock the boat or deviate in any significant way. The incident-reporting mechanism is a common example. If an employee reports making a mistake, a familiar response is for the manager to determine what went wrong and how the employee needs to change so that the mistake never occurs again—a return to the status quo. Less frequent is a response that investigates the mistake in partnership with employees to determine why the mistake occurred and what needs to change in the system so that the problem does not occur again. Recent emphasis on patient safety and the quality process has stimulated a move toward more creative problem solving and resolution without placing blame.

Leaders are always looking for ways to improve the current situation; they are never satisfied with the status quo. A leader's automatic response to a problem or mistake is to consider ways to capitalize on the opportunity that the mistake has created. For this reason, Bennis points out, "bureaucracies tend to suppress real leadership because real leaders disequilibrate systems; they create disorder and instability, even chaos" (Flower, 1990, p. 62).

Because a leader trusts people, he or she knows that the follower can always find a way to improve on the current situation. DePree (1989) describes highly effective leaders as those who are comfortable abandoning themselves to others' strengths and admitting that they themselves cannot know or do everything. This can be frightening to those who are not up to the challenge of continually questioning their own performance or established practices. Fearful individuals may react to this drive for continual improvement as implied criticism: "It was not good enough, and now we have to change it."

Bottom Line Versus Horizon

Managers keep their eyes on the bottom line; leaders focus on the horizon. Managers ask: Are we within budget? Are we meeting our goals? What's the deadline? The manager's emphasis is on counting, recording, and measuring to ensure that everything is on target. It is easy to forget that many things that count—that are important—cannot be counted.

By its very nature, leadership and its results are difficult to measure. How do you measure a relationship? What are the concrete, observable outcomes of a healthy working relationship? How do you evaluate the success of an inspiring vision? Good leaders see beyond the bottom line to the horizon, where a vision of a different future for themselves and their followers guides their day-to-day decision making. This vision inspires them to make very difficult decisions on behalf of the organization and the people within it.

A leader with a vision of empowered employees who feel ownership of their jobs, who make decisions affecting work in their span of control, and who work in partnership with the organization's managers knows that in order to attain this vision, the employees will need continual learning opportunities. In many organizations today, employees are being asked to contribute more, learn additional skills, and take on more responsibility at the same time that their organizations have severely reduced education departments and learning resources. Leadership decisions to invest in employee education may not look good on the bottom line, but they are at the core of the vision of the future. Exemplary leaders recognize that organizations that do not invest in the development of internal staff resources now will have to pay a much higher price in the future.

Another simple example of the difference between focusing on results and paying attention to the future payoff is evident when we observe leaders who become actively involved in coaching their employees for improved performance. If an employee is having difficulty with a key vendor, people in another department, or perhaps a physician, a manager may tend to use his or her legitimate authority to solve the problem. Coaching and supporting the employee in solving the problem directly may be more time-consuming and riskier. However, this leadership approach creates stronger, more effective employees; and the payoff is in the future because employees learn how to handle their own problems.

Management Versus Leadership: A Final Word

That there is a difference between management and leadership is clear. None of this is to imply, however, that there is not a need for good, capable managers in today's health care organizations. Managers will always be needed, and the role is so crucial that everyone in the organization must share managerial responsibilities. Highly efficient employees who understand their work, who are able to organize and structure it, and who can measure outcomes and take corrective action will always be in high demand. With a greater number of experienced and mature workers in health care today, organizations place higher expectations of employees than ever before. As more employees become self-managing, organizations may reduce the number of formal managers. At the same time, however, there is an increasing need for leaders. According to many recognized students of U.S. leadership, organizations in this country have been over-managed and underled (Bennis and Nanus, 1985; Kouzes and Posner, 2002; Peters, 1987).

Why Leadership Is in Demand Today

During the 1970s health care organizations had a burgeoning interest in management development programs. Recognition that promoting technically competent employees into management positions produced a responsibility on the part of the organization to provide management and supervisory training and education. In the 1990s there was a shift in all sectors of our society to emphasize the importance of leadership skills. The number of titles about leadership in a popular bookstore reflects this emphasis. A search on amazon.com produces over seventy-eight thousand hits; and when the search is narrowed to health care, the hits number over fifty-four thousand. Why this focus on leadership? Why the need to differentiate it from management? There are at least three major reasons:

- The unrelenting crush of change

- Rapidly shifting paradigms

- Survival

Change

Change has been the byword since the early 1990s, for almost fifteen years. Never has the pace of change been so fast, nor have the changes altered so deeply the way people live and work. "The change and upheaval of the past years have left us with no place to hide. We need anchors in our lives, something like a trim-tab factor, a guiding purpose. Leaders fill that need" (Bennis, 1989, p. 15). Fundamental changes in health care are occurring so rapidly that it is hard to keep pace. What we all believed to be significant organizational changes in the 1980s—revised job descriptions, new management positions, novel performance appraisals—pale by comparison to today's changes, such as new locations for services, specialty or niche hospitals, distance medicine, virtual patients, health care on the Internet, replacing employees by automation, outsourcing, cross training of skills, forming partnerships within the community, simultaneously collaborating and competing with the same entity, and merging with other organizations or developing an entirely new system. Annison (1994, p. 1) states the case clearly: "During periods of stability we can be successful by doing more of what we already do; the focus is on management and maintaining the present. During periods of change, the emphasis is on changing what we do and the focus is on leadership."

Shifting Paradigms

Paradigms, or the models through which we view the world, are rapidly shifting. Barker (1992, p. 37) describes it this way: "A paradigm shift, then, is a change to a new game, a new set of rules." This shift creates confusion and unease as well as new possibilities. In some instances, a player in the health care sector changes the paradigm, whereas in other situations the impetus comes from without. The rules and game plan may suddenly change, leaving those in the game to figure out the new rules.

Competition in health care is a good example of a paradigm that continues to shift. Not so long ago, the major competitor for a hospital was the other hospital in town, just down the road. Today competition comes from everywhere: stand-alone health care facilities, such as ambulatory-care centers, specialty hospitals and services, and diagnostic centers in physician offices; hospitals from other communities that set up satellite or full-service facilities outside their originating communities; and even previous customers who decide to become providers on a limited basis.

The lines and boundaries are no longer clear. As the business world has demonstrated, one must sometimes collaborate with close competitors (Annison, 1997). Consumers buying an Apple computer may be purchasing a machine manufactured by Toshiba; MasterCard and Visa collaborate on automatic teller machines and choose to compete on marketing and customer service. Similarly, in health care, two hospitals from competing systems have jointly built a wellness facility in their community; and a major medical center has partnered with a large clinic-based physician practice on several joint projects while competing with it on several others.

Times of great change and rapidly shifting paradigms call for leaders. As Barker (1992, p. 164) points out: "You manage within a paradigm. You lead between paradigms." When times are stable and game rules remain consistent and known, structures, standards, and protocols enhance the manager's ability to optimize the paradigm. In fact, this describes the manager's job exactly. However, during a shift to new paradigms, leadership is required, as Barker explains: "Leaving one paradigm while it is still successful and going to a new paradigm that is as yet unproved looks very risky. But leaders, with their intuitive judgment, assess the seeming risk, determine that shifting paradigms is the correct thing to do, and, because they are leaders, instill the courage in others to follow them" (p. 164).

When paradigms shift and the rules change, everyone involved goes back to zero. Put simply in the words of a colleague: "What got you to the party won't keep you there!" It is time to let go of past successes and look for new ways of doing things. There is no guarantee that the organization, group, or individual that was very good with the old game rules will be as good with the new ones. In fact, the more successful the individual or organization was with the old model, the more difficult it is to engage in a new way of thinking.

One of the major leadership gaps that market research for this book identified was a refusal to let go of the hospital mentality and traditional modes of service. Potential consequences of this pitfall include the following:

Belief that past or current success automatically leads to future success

Reluctance to make changes rapidly enough to successfully adapt to the changing external environment

Overreliance on internal expertise and past experience

Aversion to risk sharing with physicians and key stakeholders and risk taking by executives and board members

Attempts to control and dictate community health initiatives rather than collaborate with community stakeholders

This issue is easy to talk about but difficult to deal with when we are faced with a shifted paradigm. During a team retreat for surgical services leaders, initial discussion revolved around changes the team and service were experiencing. The anesthesiologists were especially upset because, with increasing managed-care penetration in their community, surgery was for the first time being considered a cost center rather than a revenue source for the organization. In their words, "We used to be able to get whatever we wanted; now we're being seen as a drain on the resources of the organization." This leadership team needed to figure out how to be successful with the new game rules in order to continue to thrive.

Survival

The final and perhaps most important reason that we need leadership today is simply survival. Bennis (1989) reported the work of a scientist at the University of Michigan who examined and listed what he considered to be the ten basic dangers to our society, factors that he believed were capable of destroying the human species. The top three are

A nuclear war or accident, capable of destroying the human race

A worldwide epidemic, disease, famine, or financial depression

The quality of management and leadership in our institutions

There was probably no clearer example of the importance of leadership in our world as during the immediate aftermath of the devastating terrorist attacks in this country on 9/11. The actions and decisions of our national leaders were crucial. Hasty and reactive actions could have led to even more devastating results. The quality and importance of leaders who emerged was striking.

Leaders are responsible for an organization's effectiveness. As an industry, health care is vulnerable as a result of regulatory changes, technological pressures, globalization, the litigious mind-set, changing demographics, and environmental challenges. Strong leadership is needed to take us into a very uncertain future. Pinchot and Pinchot (1996a, p. 18) eloquently describe the need for leaders: "The more machines take over routine work and the higher the percentage of knowledge workers, the more leaders are needed. The work left for humans involves innovation, seeing things in new ways, and responding to customers by changing the way things are done. We are reaching a time when every employee will take turns leading. Each will find circumstances when they see what must be done and must influence others to make their vision of a better way a reality."

Finally, the role of leaders as it influences organizations' integrity is crucial. "There is a pervasive, national concern about the integrity of our institutions. Wall Street was, not long ago, a place where a man's word was his bond. The recent investigations, revelations, and indictments have forced the industry to change the way it conducted business for 150 years. Jim Bakker and Jimmy Swaggart have given a new meaning to the phrase 'children of a lesser God' " (Bennis, 1989, pp. 15–16). Although Bennis wrote those words years ago, they seem almost prophetic. In the last few years, Americans have become almost inured to corporate scandal and wrongdoing. The collapse of Enron, Arthur Andersen, and WorldCom are just samples in what seems to be a never-ending parade of corporate corruption. Many Americans now fully expect that people in leadership positions who lack personal and professional integrity will lie and cheat.

Health care is not immune to the issue of integrity. Hospital executives indicted for Medicare fraud, home health agencies led by criminals previously convicted of fraud, a cardiovascular surgeon falsifying information and performing hundreds of clearly unnecessary surgeries, a pharmacist diluting chemotherapeutic agents to increase profit, executives at a well-known rehabilitation company indicted for illegal practices, or a community hospital's senior executives convicted of embezzlement—all have made the headlines in recent years. Never has the need for ethical, exemplary leaders been more crucial as we face the challenges of the next century.

Challenges Facing Today's Leaders

Today the opportunities and possibilities for leaders are endless, as are the challenges. Demands are different for today's leaders and have ramifications for anyone aspiring to lead others. The more a leader understands these issues, the more likely he or she can find the necessary strength and courage to meet the test that these challenges present:

- The rapidity of change
- Workforce shortages
- The rise of the free-agent mentality

- Diversity in the workforce

- New organizational structures

- Turbulent business environments

- The leader's energy capacity

The Rapidity of Change

Change is occurring at an accelerated pace today, and change experts assure the public that the rate of change will continue to increase through the end of this decade. According to Connor (1993, p. 39), change in previous eras was different in magnitude and pace, the approach required, the increasing seriousness of its implication, and the short shelf life of solutions: "In tumultuous environments, every solution brings more complex problems, not worse necessarily, but ones requiring more creative approaches. For example, the world is not worse off because of the invention of the computer. But even with all the good that these machines have provided, information systems have complicated our lives in unforeseen ways." It can be discouraging when a leader realizes that today's solution may become tomorrow's problem. Leaders know that the current change simply brings you closer to the next one.

Change takes energy; and as we experience more change, it can feel like an endless energy drain. Because influencing others positively when we are exhausted is difficult, leaders must take good care of themselves during changing times and manage their energy wisely (Loehr and Schwartz, 2003; Cox, Manion, and Miller, 2005). Not all changes are for the better, and a leader is challenged to remain optimistic and enthusiastic yet truthful. This can be arduous in the face of personal discouragement. As Connor (1993) describes it, effective leaders have a high degree of resilience in their ability to demonstrate courage, strength, and flexibility in the face of change and frightening disorder.

Sometimes the challenge for a leader lies in determining which changes to make and which to forgo. It is easy to become swept up in the tide of change and go overboard. Many leaders find change exhilarating and forget that the organization's ability to sustain a certain pace of change may not match the leader's capacity for change. Winston Churchill said, "When it is not necessary to change, it is necessary not to change" (Curtin, 1995, p. 7). This sage advice is easy to forget when all the changes look positive. The knack of looking beyond the initial excitement and potential promise to determine whether the change is necessary and beneficial is a leadership skill worth developing.

A community hospital undergoing a major restructuring and work-redesign effort provided an unintended example of this tendency to get caught up in unnecessary change. As the hospital restructured departments, management asked clinical employees to reapply for their positions. There was concern that the secretaries and executive assistants in the organization would not have the same opportunity (yes, it was considered an opportunity). As a result, all employees in secretarial positions were allowed to apply for a transfer into any position for which they were suited. The outcome was an extreme version of "fruit basket upset." The secretary for the behavioral health department transferred to education; the education secretary went to human resources; the human resource secretary transferred to purchasing; the infection control secretary went to administration; and so on. The result was mass confusion and significantly decreased effectiveness in the organization for a good six months while these people were being oriented—all for what was, in the end, unnecessary change.

Peter Drucker talks about this same issue (Flower, 1991, p. 53), but he refers to it as being effective. He says the leader has to sometimes say no: "The secret of effectiveness is concentration of the very meager resources you have where you can make a difference." Thus, the leader's role is to carefully assess what changes are most important and likely to help achieve the organization's goals and attain its vision while avoiding the energy drain of nonessential change.

Every major sector of society is undergoing massive change. The entire structure of health care is changing. A book edited by Chawla and Renesch (1995) found factors at work requiring critical shifts in thinking by health care leaders, factors such as the following:

A shift from fee-for-service to discounts and capitation, in which providers are responsible for quality and cost

A shift from inpatient acute-care to outpatient services, requiring health care leaders to rethink traditional hospital boundaries, investments, and relationships with key stakeholders

The rise of primary care physicians as gatekeepers and care managers in a capitated environment

A shift from a discipline-centered production organization to a customer-focused service orientation

A shift from an illness and disease model to a wellness paradigm with a focus on alternative or complementary medicine

Along with this challenge is the fact that many people are in transition. The word *change* means to alter or make something different. *Transition* is the psychological adaptation to change and is not over until the person can function and find meaning in the new situation (Bridges, 1991). If a transition has occurred, something has been lost, even if it is as simple as loss of comfort with the old way. Thus, stages of transition include stages of grief, which engender some of the most difficult emotions humans face. People often experience and express anger, depression, anxiety, fear, and just plain contrariness. Trying to lead people who are grieving is fraught with difficulties and can tax even the most proficient leader.

These emotions are complex enough to face in an individual, much less when multiplied by hundreds and even thousands in an organization. Understanding where people are in their emotional cycle helps prevent inappropriate or unhelpful responses. The fact that they may all be in different places at the same time makes the challenge more intense. Adding to the complexity is the fact that the leader may be feeling some of these difficult emotions as well. Chapter Five explores the transition process in more detail.

Workforce Shortages

The large number of baby boomers nearing retirement age and the declining numbers of younger workers entering health care is rapidly reaching a crisis point. This challenge is surfacing as one of the most difficult in this decade and is likely to remain a paramount concern for many years into the future. A poll of hospital CEOs by the American Hospital Association (2001) found that 72 percent of respondents identified workforce shortages as one of the top three concerns. Demographics alone tell us that workforce shortages are not just a temporary challenge but part of the landscape for many years to come.

"Never before have organizations paid more attention to talent . . . keeping it. Stealing it. Developing it. Engaging it. Talent is no longer just a numbers game; it's about survival" (Kaye and Jordan-Evans, 2002, p. 32). Workforce shortage issues are not limited to one discipline nor one job category in our organizations but cut across all boundaries. Although the literature often focuses on the cost of turnover of higher-paid professionals such as pharmacists, nurses, and physical therapists, a significant cost is also associated with the turnover and vacancy of workers in positions such as housekeepers, dietary aides, and nursing assistants. This cost may be lower per individual, but the sheer number of these workers employed in the average health care organization makes the cost almost prohibitive. A recent study of long-term care organizations reported turnover rates of nurse aides near 100 percent annually. This represents a tremendous cost to the organization, one that far exceeds the financial impact.

The stability and quality of the workforce is directly linked to better outcomes and higher-quality services in our organizations (Aiken, Clarke, and Stone, 2002; American Hospital Association,

2001; Batcheller and others, 2004; Gelinas and Bohlen, 2002; Unruh, 2004). Although recruitment of talented individuals into health care is an important strategy, it is clearly not adequate. Not only are pools of possible workers smaller, but the competition is greater because of the wide variety of career and vocational options that are available to people today. Health care no longer offers the same level of security that it did in the past. In addition to the loss of job security, safety concerns and stress are major issues today (American Nurses Association, 2001; AbuAlRub, 2004).

The challenge for today's health care leader is to create positive work environments that not only attract high-quality candidates but retain them. And although people seldom join an organization today with the intent of remaining in its employment throughout their career, simply extending the length of tenure of high-quality employees by several years can have a positive impact on vacancy and turnover rates.

The Rise of the Free-Agent Mentality

In the earliest days of modern organized health care, hospitals operated with student nurses and perhaps a limited number of professional nurses. Other specialized workers did not exist. Patients or their families employed graduate nurses as independent contractors. They functioned as free agents rather than as employees of the organization.

This mirrors a fundamental shift in work life that is occurring across the United States today and affecting people in unexpected ways. The shift is away from the job as a concept. William Bridges, author of several best-selling books, including *Transitions*, *Managing Transitions*, and *Surviving Corporate Transition*, describes this concept in his book *JobShift* (1994a). He notes that the concept of a job was only invented at the beginning of the industrial revolution, when people went to work in factories. With the decline of manufacturing and the evolution of the information age, the very concept of the job as we knew it is disintegrating.

"As a way of organizing work, [the job] is a social artifact that has outlived its usefulness. Its demise confronts everyone with unfamiliar risks—and rich opportunities" (Bridges, 1994b, p. 62). This trend is disturbing to many people who have remained in a long-term employment setting their entire work life. It is difficult to conceive of a dejobbed health care organization, and yet many examples are already apparent. With growing workforce shortages and the increasingly stiff competition between organizations for qualified employees, health care workers are more likely to move among organizations for their employment. There is an increase in outsourcing and use of consultants and independent contractors. Part-timers outnumber full-time employees in some organizations; it's not uncommon to have employees with two to three jobs; and the consistent use of per diem or registry staff is expanding to disciplines beyond nursing. These are all examples that support this trend toward dejobbing health care.

Although it is unlikely that health care will ever be completely dejobbed (Flower, 1997), this trend does have implications for leaders. "The main impact is . . . that tomorrow's leadership is going to have to be able to activate and focus the efforts of people who lack long-term connections with or loyalty to the organization. You don't lead a group of freelancers the way you lead long-term employees" (Bridges, 1995, p. 5). Influencing these people and getting commitment from them is much tougher than when the employees' connections to the organization were stronger.

Closely related to the dejobbing challenge yet somewhat different is the altered contract that organizations have with their employees. Not so very long ago, when an institution hired employees, the implication—and reality—of the agreement was that as long as the employee completed work according to expected standards, the employee retained the job. Even in the face of economic downturns, health care workers enjoyed fairly high job security. Not so anymore. There are no longer guarantees of any kind but instead what author David Noer (1993, p. 13) describes as a new employment contract: "This psychological contract fits the new reality. It says that even the best performer or the most culturally adaptive person cannot count on long-term employment. It replaces loyalty to an organization with loyalty to one's work."

Examples of this abound in health care since the early 1990s. Even employees with long-term employment in an organization have found themselves suddenly and inexplicably out of a job. In one case, a director of staff development attended a professional seminar on a Friday; the topic was dealing with change in the workplace. When she returned to work the following Monday, she learned that she needed to decide by noon which two employees she would choose to eliminate or lay off. At one o'clock she learned that she would be reporting directly to the vice president of human resources because the director of education (to whom she usually reported) had been eliminated. None of these employees was doing a bad job; the organization had simply eliminated the positions because it had experienced a significant financial downturn and viewed these job cuts as a way to reduce expenses.

Another organization eliminated several long-term, excellent employees when it outsourced their function in the human resource department. In yet another organization, the vice president of human resources helped lead the "rightsizing" campaign—only to discover that the last position to be eliminated was his own! In the 1990s many organizations consolidated management positions and eliminated people even though they were contributing and highly committed employees. Entire categories of positions were eliminated, such as supervisors, clinical nurse specialists, lead technicians, assistant managers, clinicians, and charge nurses, to cite a few examples.

Not all of these changes were bad; perhaps they reflected the beginning of a transition to a more fluid, flexible organization of the future. However, the end result is a clear understanding within the hearts of health care workers that the job is not sacred, that they too can be eliminated at the whim of organizational need. And fortunately or unfortunately, many of these organizations found that you can eliminate people much more easily than the actual work; and they have since found it necessary to reinstate these or similar positions. All this leaves employees questioning whether leaders actually know what they are doing when they make some of these sweeping decisions.

This disruption in employment can also be healthy for the in-dustry as a whole. Noer (1993) believes that the past model sus-tained an unhealthy, outdated organizational codependency. It was not unusual for employees to depend on the organization for far more than a job or a way to earn a living. It was similar to the old company store mentality, and employees expected the organization to provide everything: a network of friends, a social life, recreational opportunities, education support, and health care benefits.

"This battle is among the most important struggles that we and our organizations have ever faced. Individuals must break the chains of their unhealthy, outdated organizational codependency and recapture their self-esteem; organizations must achieve their poten-tial and thrive in the new world economy. For the organization, holding on to the familiar old is not the answer" (Noer, 1993, p. 4). And, for the individual, holding onto the job is not always the healthiest option.

Noer's advice (1993, p. 15) is striking: "The only way you pro-vide security for yourself is by making sure that your work experi-ence is as up-to-date as possible so that if tomorrow happens, you are able to go out and get another job because you have skills peo-ple want. That's the only way you have security. You aren't going to get it from the company. It will never be that way again." He per-fectly describes the free-agent mentality that the health care employee needs today.

This new employment contract has significant ramifications for health care leaders. These chains of organizational codependency can be as difficult to break for those who have provided these benefits and implied job security as for those who have been the recipients of the supposed rewards. Many leaders still feel benevolence toward employ-ees and do not want to accept that a healthier relationship is a full partnership between the employee and the organization. The generosity of the "we will take care of you" attitude has inadvertently created employees who are overly dependent on the organization. And as organizations reduce benefits and talk less of the "big, happy family," employees naturally respond as if organizations are taking away what the employees had felt entitled to.

Diversity in the Workforce

When anyone asks health care leaders what their greatest challenges are today, increasing diversity in the workplace is almost always at the top of the list. As a leader in a recent program noted, "In our organization there are sixty-five different languages spoken." The globalization of our world has certainly made an impact in the workplace in terms of the various cultures and ethnic groups of the people who work together. However, this is not the only diversity creating increased challenges for leaders. Never before has there been such diversity in workers' ages. The health care workforce employs large numbers of women, and the baby boomers reaching retirement age are the first generation of women who entered and remained in the workforce throughout an entire career.

Additionally, although we have always been aware that the generations differ in attitudes and beliefs, friction between members of these age cohorts seems to be accelerating. Furthermore, there is a suggestion that the time required to produce significant differences between age groups is compressing; whereas our grandparents were markedly different from our parents and from us, now there are significant differences between three siblings, ages twenty-one, eighteen, and fifteen (Maun, 2004). This stems directly from the rapidity of world changes we are experiencing in this very tumultuous environment.

The challenge for the health care leader can feel overwhelming at times. How can one person lead such a diverse group of employees who are providing service and care to an even more widely diverse group of patients and families? How can we benefit from the creativity and opportunity that such diversity represents while respecting the many differences and not allowing relationships to degenerate into unmanageable conflict and confusion?

New Organizational Structures

We need new organizational structures to meet the demands of changing times. The transition from a resident-based to a mobility-based model of care (Porter-O'Grady and Malloch, 2003) requires a more fluid and dynamic organizational model. This is a major challenge given that most of today's leaders have spent the majority of their organizational life in a bureaucratic structure, one with which they are comfortable. Whether this structure can survive into the future is debatable.

In the 1990s organizations tried new, more fluid and flexible structures with the belief that these newer structures would enhance response to customers, increase the rate of innovation, and create work environments that stimulate employee commitment, curiosity, and ownership. In their book *The Intelligent Organization*, Pinchot and Pinchot (1996b, p. xiv) write: "The transformation from bureaucracy to organizational intelligence is a move from relationships of dominance and submission up and down the chain of command to horizontal relationships of peers across a network of voluntary cooperation and market-based exchanges."

Leadership scholars have been pointing out for years that bureaucracies are not well equipped to meet changing times. Bennis notes, "Bureaucracies are self-sustaining only in times of stability, when the environment is placid. They are very ineffective when times are changing. When the world is turbulent, the managerial environment is spastic, fluid, and volatile. Then the bureaucracy seems to be particularly inadequate because it keeps repeating yesterday's lessons and fighting the last war" (Flower, 1990, p. 62). Organizations of the future are more likely to be based on a network or a flattened hierarchy model. In fact, Bennis is very clear on this point when he says in the same interview, "Organizations that operate on the nineteenth-century model of the bureaucracy—a model based on the words control, order, and predict—are just not going to cut it. . . . They already aren't" (Flower, 1990, p. 62).

One new form of organizational model is what Waterman (1992) called the adhocracy, which is any organizational form that challenges the bureaucracy in order to embrace new ways of doing things. He notes that the concept of adhocracy is not new. In the mid-1960s, he writes (p. 18), "Warren Bennis argued the need for adaptive, problem-solving, temporary systems of diverse specialists linked together . . . in an organic flux." This is much more difficult to do in a bureaucracy than it appears. People hold specific jobs and have responsibilities that must be accomplished regardless of temporary assignments or project team commitments. Health care during the 1990s saw more of a move toward flexible assignments than was in evidence prior to this time. When undergoing major reengineering or work-redesign initiatives, many organizations appointed employees or managers as project directors or project team members. This pulled employees and managers out of their jobs and moved them into these semipermanent yet temporary assignments. It allowed organizations to move some of their best and brightest people to the critical initiative of the day.

This resulted in many other difficulties, however, the prime predicament being what to do with these people when they had completed the temporary work and the organization had filled or eliminated the individual's previous job. It is the same problem in other businesses and industries, as Waterman (1992, p. 26) notes: "Today's companies need, but seldom have, the ability to move seamlessly from bureaucracy to adhocracy and back again. Today's managers need, but seldom have, the skill and security to leave their posts for a while and become effective members of project teams. But without that ability, companies and people go on making the same old mistakes. They do not learn. This is the Achilles' heel of corporate America." This remains an issue in today's health care organizations. Some larger systems may be more flexible in creating roles designed to take on current initiatives; however, financial constraints have severely limited resources in most organizations, which do not have the luxury of being flexible.

Another promising organizational form attempted in the 1990s was the team-based organization. This structure "replaces or supplements traditional hierarchical structures with semiautonomous teams in order to flatten management, revitalize employees, and enhance productivity" (Manion, Lorimer, and Leander, 1996, p. xi). Many organizations attempted to create employee work teams that replaced the department as the smallest unit of an organization's structure. Teams were touted as a way to forge a partnership between leaders and employees, capable of producing an undreamed-of synergy as teams built on the strengths of everyone in the organization. Unfortunately, few organizations were able to truly convert their systems to a team-based structure; and most organizations that made the attempt have only remnants of the structure remaining today. Although a team-based structure offered a possibility for softening the bureaucratic, hierarchical structure of a health care organization, it simply did not materialize in most organizations. The true essence of teams involves transfer of real responsibility and authority to the team and formation of a collaborative relationship between manager and team. Creating a true team-based organization challenges both leadership skills and beliefs. It simply cannot occur without strong leaders who have a clear vision of a different future and are willing to share power.

Shared decision-making models are similar in concept and more accurately describe current work aimed at modifying the organizational bureaucracy. These approaches are based on the belief that those who are closest to the work should be involved in the decisions affecting that work. Organizations espousing this belief establish structures that enhance employee participation in decision making.

Turbulent Business Environment

The business environment within which health care organizations exist is tumultuous and unpredictable. Declining levels of reimbursement, increasing costs of products and materials, the availability of Internet-based health care, the litigious mind-set, the appearance of watchdog groups focused on patient outcomes and safety, escalating workforce shortages and worker demands, increasing competition from physicians, and the demands of increasing regulation all serve to create uncertainty in the health care marketplace. These create tremendous challenges as well as opportunities for leaders. Struggling to stay one step ahead requires leaders to spend tremendous energy and renew their commitment day to day and sometimes even hour to hour.

A story illustrates this challenge perfectly. In Africa each day a lion wakes up. He knows he will need to outrun the fastest gazelle if he is to eat that day. Each day in Africa, a gazelle wakes up and knows he will need to outrun the fastest lion if he is to stay alive that day. The moral: it does not matter if you are a lion or a gazelle, as long as you wake up running! Translated for health care: every leader must wake up ready to face these challenges every single day, or we will fall behind.

The rapidity with which our business environment can change became evident in the late 1990s. One home health agency lost over 60 percent of its reimbursed business overnight with a change in the reimbursement of phlebotomy. Hospitals with healthy bottom lines experienced severe reversals in their financial picture within months due to unanticipated reimbursement changes. The financial health of today's health care organizations can best be described as highly volatile.

The Leader's Energy Capacity

In light of these challenges, or perhaps as a result of these issues, health care leaders face the personal challenge of maintaining and expanding their own energy capacity. This is likely the ultimate leadership challenge of this decade. In the face of increasing demands and escalating complexity in our environment and work, how do I as a leader locate and protect my sources of personal energy? And perhaps more important, how do I increase my capacity in order to deal with these multiple challenges?

Health care leaders not only have permission to care for themselves, they have a responsibility to do so (Collins, 1992). When you think of the tremendous national resource of our outstanding leaders and managers, they are indeed a precious asset. Often these leaders come from the ranks of people who started their career in service to others or as caregivers. Self-care may not come naturally to those who have spent their life in service to others. As Collins (p. 5) writes, "Caring for others is a hazardous occupation . . . those of us who care for others have trouble caring for ourselves."

Everything we do consumes energy. Understanding the flow of energy within a system, whether the organization or the self, is a way to increase our proficiency at managing energy and ultimately increasing our capacity (Cox, Manion, and Miller, 2005). Loehr and Schwartz (2003) believe that managing our energy is the key to high performance and personal self-renewal, not becoming increasingly proficient at managing time. Finding and keeping a reasonable balance between our work, family, and personal worlds is a remarkable yet crucial feat for today's organizational leader (Bowcutt, 2004; Fields and Zwisler, 2004; Larson and William, 2004; Ulreich, 2004; Van Allen, 2004).

Conclusion

Developing leaders is one of the most important issues currently facing health care organizations. In defining leadership, it is important to distinguish between leadership and management. The growing need for strong leadership is directly related to the unrelenting crush of change we experience today, which in the health care world is reflected in the rapid shifting of paradigms and concern for survival into the future. The many challenges facing today's leaders are closely intertwined and interdependent. They include the rapidity of change, workforce shortages, the free-agent mentality, increasing diversity in the workplace, the need for new organizational structures, the tumultuous business environment, and the need for managing one's own energy capacity. These factors have resulted in a tremendous sense of urgency in health care organizations and have made clear the need for the identification and development of internal leaders as well as the mastery of new, nontraditional skills for these leaders.

Conversation Points

1. Think about people who have been effective leaders in your life. How did their behaviors compare to the description of leadership that this chapter offered?

2. What does your organization emphasize—leadership or management? Consider carefully both the verbal and the behavioral messages from established organizational leaders.

3. Think about your own skills. Where do your strengths fall? Are you a stronger leader or a stronger manager? Where do you have opportunities for improvement? Do you need to change your mix of skills?

4. Think about the person to whom you report. Where do that person's strongest skills lie: in management or leadership? What kind of impact does this have on you?

5. What are your biggest challenges as a leader today? If you are not currently functioning as a leader, what are the biggest challenges that leaders in your organization, religious organization, community, or our country face today?

2

Cultivating the
Leadership Relationship

The only definition of a leader is someone who has
followers.
Some people are thinkers. Some are prophets. Both
roles are important and badly needed.
But without followers, there can be no leaders.

Peter Drucker, Managing for the Future

Leadership exists only within the context of a relationship. It is an intensely personal experience, a process of relating to another person, who, if influenced, becomes a follower. All definitions of leadership include the ability to influence others to do what needs to be done. It is a dynamic interaction between leader and follower, changing each irrevocably.

The emphasis on the importance of the relationship between the leader and the follower has become evident in recent years. Research in the area of emotional intelligence clearly demonstrates that the emotions of the leader directly affect the atmosphere and quality of the leader's relationships with others (Goleman, 1994; Goleman, Boyatzis, and McKee, 2002). The emotionally intelligent leader is one who is able "to generate excitement, optimism, and passion for the job ahead, as well as to cultivate an atmosphere of cooperation and trust" (Goleman, Boyatzis, and McKee, 2002, p. 29). These leaders need competencies in four different domains:

self-awareness, self-management, social awareness, and relationship management. Figure 2.1 presents these four domains as well as the competencies that exist within them. Closely intertwined, these competencies form the basis of effectiveness in the workplace.

An early definition of *emotional intelligence* was "The ability to perceive and express emotion, assimilate emotion in thought, understand and reason with emotion, and regulate emotion in the self and others" (Mayer, Salovey, and Caruso, 2000, p. 396). This means that the leader has a high degree of self-awareness and is able to recognize his or her own emotion accurately. Not only is this self-awareness

	Self (Personal competence)	Other (Social competence)
Recognition	Self-Awareness Emotional self-awareness Accurate self-assessment Self-confidence	Social Awareness Empathy Service orientation Organizational awareness
Regulation	Self-Management Emotional self-control Trustworthiness Conscientiousness Adaptability Achievement drive Initiative	Relationship Management Developing others Influence Communication Conflict management Visionary leadership Catalyzing change Building bonds Teamwork and collaboration

Figure 2.1. Emotional Intelligence Competencies

Source: The Emotionally Intelligent Workplace © 2001. Reprinted with permission of John Wiley & Sons, Inc., Hoboken, N.J.

accurate, but importantly, the individual is able to regulate a response to the emotion. Here's a clear example: several department employees confronted a manager. The employees were very angry about a recent administrative decision. They confronted their manager by saying, "We're surprised you aren't angry about this, what's the matter with you?" The leader took them by surprise when she replied, "Oh, do not mistake me, I am very angry about this. But I don't need to let that anger erupt all over everyone here. I can control it." And her brief words gave the employees a beautiful role model of an emotionally intelligent leader capable of regulating her emotions.

But emotional intelligence is not limited to the individual level. The leader also is competent in relationships with others, both in social awareness as well as in relationship management. These build on the personal competencies of recognition (emotional self-awareness, accurate self-assessment, and self-confidence) as well as self-regulation (emotional self-control, trustworthiness, conscientiousness, adaptability, achievement drive, and initiative). The social competencies related to social awareness include empathy, a service orientation, and an organizational awareness (Cherniss and Goleman, 2001). Other authors and scholars have identified the importance of these competencies as well. "The caring part of empathy, especially for the people with whom you work, is what inspires people to stay with a leader when the going gets rough. The mere fact that someone cares is more often than not rewarded with loyalty" (Champy, 2003, p. 135).

The quality of the leader and follower's relationship directly affects the leader's abilities. Without the foundation for a healthy relationship, the aspiring leader cannot attain extraordinary outcomes. Although troubled leaders seldom return to the basic components of a healthy relationship when they are frustrated by followers who do not follow, the answer to their difficulties often lies within this basic concept. This chapter outlines the essential elements of a healthy leader-follower relationship and identifies several future-oriented forms of association that today's leaders must understand.

Essential Elements of a Healthy Relationship

Leaders who relate comfortably to others often take for granted their talent for forming relationships. Their relationships have a natural-ness and a spontaneity that result in mutually beneficial outcomes. When a particular leader-follower situation is not going well, the relationship-centered leader often reflects first on the connection with the supporter to determine the issues. And because this leader is already skillful in this area, the assessment process is not likely to produce undue anxiety. But if the leader is not naturally talented at forming strong relationships, this affects both the accuracy and ease of the assessment process. However, one can increase one's skills in this area.

Established, effective leaders often intuitively understand the es-sential elements of a healthy relationship. And when something is wrong, intuitive signals alert the leader. There are at least three es-sential elements of a successful leader-follower relationship:

- Trust

- Mutual respect

- Communication

These three elements are essential because the absence of any one can damage the relationship.

Trust

According to *Webster's Encyclopedic Unabridged Dictionary*, *trust* means you can rely on the "integrity, strength or ability of a person or thing. Confidence implies conscious trust because of good reasons, definite evidence or past experience." Without trust or confidence in the person attempting to influence them, people will not follow that person's direction or lead. In an organization, when the in-dividual attempting to lead relies primarily on the legitimate authority of his or her position, the relative health of the relationship can be deceptive. People may do what that leader wants not because they agree or believe in the direction the leader sets or the request he or she makes, but because they believe they must comply or suffer painful or undesirable consequences.

Understanding the concept of trust is imperative for anyone aspiring to lead others. Warren Bennis (Flower, 1990) offers a concrete, applicable framework for understanding trust within the context of a leadership role. He defines three essential ingredients for trust as competence, congruence, and constancy. Examining these three components of trust provides a guide for any leader who is seeking to more fully understand his or her personal effectiveness.

Competence

Webster's defines *competence* as the "possession of required skill, knowledge, qualification or capacity." The application of this definition in a leadership context is clear. Supporters must believe that the leader has the skill and knowledge to do what is required. "Whenever we step in front of the crowd and say, 'Follow me,' the implication is that we know where we're going and what we want to achieve and that we're committed to giving our very best efforts" (Melrose, 1996, p. 20). Confidence in a leader develops from working with that person and from seeing evidence of the leader's past performance demonstrating competence. Both skill and knowledge are included in this definition. Knowledge alone is insufficient. The leader may know that followers need accurate information and clear communication, but an unskilled leader who is unable to articulate clearly will be greatly hampered.

This is why changing key leaders in organizations can result in a troublesome situation. Establishing trust and confidence in new leadership takes time. Nevertheless, many health care organizations embarking on major change choose to alter the managerial and executive structure, eliminating or combining positions. Entire departments find themselves in a new reporting relationship. Leaders in these new positions are then expected to lead their followers through the changes, yet they are severely disadvantaged because they must first form a trusting relationship. Although this sequence of events may be appropriate, organizations should carefully consider the sequence's impact on the time required to create change. In one midwestern hospital, the CEO routinely changes reporting relationships every couple of years because he likes to keep people off balance, in his words, "to shake things up a bit." What he fails to see is the effect on productivity and the cost in terms of relationships.

Qualification. Qualification is an interesting factor in competence. The field of health care has a notable emphasis on expertise as a necessary qualification (as discussed in Chapter One). Some people simply do not follow an individual unless the person has a particular qualification they believe to be important, such as a clinical discipline background or a certain academic degree. Whether the qualification actually prepares or enables the leader to function competently is a moot point; to a potential follower, it can become a critical issue with significant repercussions. Organizations that have consolidated departments and replaced two or three managers with one often encounter significant obstacles when the manager no longer shares the background or expertise of the department's employees. Although this is not an insurmountable obstacle, it can take longer for the new manager to establish a trust relationship with employees because of a need to prove competence in the face of what appears to be a significant qualification issue.

Capacity. Capacity issues influence the level of trust in the leader. If others see a leader as simply having too much to do, too many responsibilities, juggling too many balls, a question of trust may arise. Can this leader handle the current situation? Will it be too much? What if it pushes the leader over the edge? A leader who appears frazzled and out of control creates uneasy followers. Personal endurance and a phenomenal capacity for work often go hand in hand with effective leadership. The motto "Never let them see you sweat" may be appropriate but should not imply that a good leader never lets followers see the reality of a difficult situation.

In one West Coast hospital undergoing significant organizational consolidation of leadership roles, a newly appointed executive had a personality style characterized by spontaneity, impulsiveness, and a high degree of self-disclosure. As the initiative progressed, this leader was given more and more responsibility because she was very capable. She quickly reached the point of overload and began manifesting counterproductive behaviors such as volatility, extreme distractibility, and pure panic. Her communication patterns became dysfunctional as a result of her intense anxiety. Her erratic behavior with her followers clearly transmitted her anxiety, and she began to lose their trust. In this instance, skill, knowledge, and qualifications were not at issue. Instead, her followers feared that she could not handle the heavy load.

Congruence

The second key element of trust in this context is congruence, meaning consistency or agreement between verbal messages and the leader's behavior (Lorimer and Manion, 1996). When what a leader says is highly congruent with what he or she does, the followers perceive the leader as honest and trustworthy. If the leader says one thing but does another, the result is an enormous credibility gap with followers. Most would agree that leaders must "walk the talk." The leader's integrity and character are important. Followers need to believe that leaders act in accordance with their personal beliefs and are honest not only with themselves but with followers. This is more important than the followers' agreeing with the leader's beliefs. "Effective leadership . . . is not based on being clever; it is based primarily on being consistent" (Drucker, 1992, p. 122).

Common Discrepancies. Examples of discrepancies are common in any work setting. One department leader in the hospital maintenance department established employee work teams and assured team members that they would have responsibility for input into decisions that would affect their work. After almost a year of working together as a team, two new team members that no one on the team had expected joined them. Their manager had hired these additional members without including the team in the decision. Consequently, the team members felt betrayed by the manager, and the ensuing breach of trust was difficult to repair. They wondered what other decisions the manager had made without their ideas or input.

One of the most serious problems with congruence is that inconsistent messages are often inadvertent. The leader usually does not purposely engage in behavior that is contrary to previous messages he or she has sent but instead, without realizing it, acts in direct contradiction to the oral and written messages delivered. This happened in one organization that stated that competence was an organization value. Yet when attempting to determine who to lay off during an economic downturn, tenure was the key selection criteria. Tenure and competence are not the same thing, and many employees were offended and angered by what appeared to be a decision-making criterion inconsistent with a stated, and often touted, organization value. When employees questioned this, the senior executive leading the initiative became defensive and angry but eventually listened to the feedback and changed the decision-making criteria. The organization then used tenure as a final determining factor only if the employees in question first met the criterion of competence.

Another hospital handled a similar situation differently. When confronted with the incongruity between the stated organization value of competence and use of tenure as a selection criterion, the administration of this community hospital retained tenure as the deciding criterion. They reasoned that this was not the appropriate time to correct problems with employee competence that managers had not dealt with previously. Though it may sound reasonable, their choice remained a major credibility issue. By saying that managers had never dealt properly with unacceptable or poor employee performance, they were basically admitting that they had never held true to the organization's stated value of competence.

Avoiding Discrepancies. A leader must scrupulously examine and be aware of behavior that others might interpret as incongruent, although avoiding all discrepancies is virtually impossible. Thus, it is especially important for a leader to promote openness and honest feedback from followers. An executive team in one northeastern medical center worked diligently to establish such an open environment, making certain that employees knew their leaders wanted feedback if their behaviors appeared incongruent. These leaders knew that their initial reaction to feedback would determine the amount and usefulness of future feedback employees would give and were very careful to listen fully and react nondefensively when employees brought discordant messages to their attention. In some instances, leaders changed behavior deemed incongruent to fit the message. In other cases, communication was unclear, and the parties resolved the problem by sharing additional information. This openness did not occur overnight. Many employees were—and some still are—hesitant to provide feedback because they feared reprisals. This fear is a common obstacle when the leader holds a hierarchical position and has legitimate power over employees.

Giving the leader feedback on incongruent behavior is much more difficult than it may appear. The majority of employees are unwilling to say anything, even if they see the leader is about to make a mistake. If their feedback is discounted by either verbal or body language, they become unwilling to speak up in the future. Some of this reluctance to speak freely and honestly is related to early socialization messages. Chaleff (1996) explains that people learn from an early age to obey authority, to say "Yes, sir" and "Yes, ma'am," and that this conditioning runs very deep. Overcoming these deep internal messages takes work. "We are afraid that if we question authority we will be viewed as a nuisance, pushed out of the loop, overlooked for promotion, even fired. We fear the consequences of speaking up far more than we are afraid of the more serious consequences of not speaking up" (p. 16).

Another way to view congruence involves congruity between what leaders do in their personal and public lives. People who do not live up to commitments to their family or who cheat their neighbors often hide behind the belief that what happens in their personal lives should not affect their leadership roles. Like it or not, if followers see untrustworthy personal behavior, this affects the level of trust they place in their leaders.

Constancy

Constancy is the third and final ingredient of trust that Bennis identified (Flower, 1990). It implies that the leader is reliable, dependable, and consistent. A good leader keeps commitments and follows through on promises made. If it becomes clear that a promise or commitment cannot be met, the leader communicates openly and honestly with followers to inform them of the changed circumstances—ideally before the followers confront the leader.

Availability and Accessibility. To many followers, availability and accessibility are part of constancy. For leaders to be most effective, they must be accessible to followers and not just at prescheduled, formal times. Some of the best dialogues occur spontaneously. When the leader is also a manager or executive, the role's formal trappings may distance the leader from followers. Common examples of this are isolated office locations or the presence of secretaries who see their role as protecting or buffering the leader from others. Although being completely available twenty-four hours a day is not possible, neither should the leader be inaccessible to followers. The leader must find a balance, for the perception that the leader is available is a potent one in creating a collegial relationship with followers.

One key way that leaders create a positive work environment is by being visible (Manion, 2004b). Peters and Austin (1985) coined the term "management by walking around," or MBWA. This suggests that the closer a leader is physically to followers, the more this establishes a sense of connection and understanding. And it is true that the leader who sees a situation with his or her own eyes is certainly better informed than one hearing about it from a third, potentially biased party. As time pressures increase, a leader often sacrifices visibility and availability. Whatever constraints may exist, they are never as serious as the threat to a leader's effectiveness from followers who do not feel a sense of connection and as a result do not follow.

These ideas seem like common sense or intuitive knowledge that is self-evident. However, availability and accessibility are difficult to achieve in these demanding times. The massive amount of change occurring creates an environment filled with uncertainty, and followers have many questions. Followers may not perceive all changes as positive and may be very unhappy, even angry, about the organization's current direction. Every leader today knows how daunting it is to face a crowd of antagonistic followers, and avoiding these situations and withdrawing from contact with followers is a natural tendency. Herein lies one major difference between the excellent leader and the not-so-effective leader: the excellent leader stays more visible and involved, more accessible and available to followers during these times. As in a sporting event in which a team finds inspiration from cheerleaders when it falls behind and is losing the game, the excellent leader knows the importance of being present when there is significant unrest. This leader understands that his or her mere presence is often a gift and message of support to uncertain followers.

Being able to count on the leader's presence is important to followers, although some leaders feel uncomfortable if they do not have answers to complex or difficult questions that followers raise. Many of today's leaders are managers, or were managers in the past, who have been socialized to believe that the manager's job is to have answers. A good leader understands and accepts, however, that having all of the answers is impossible. It takes phenomenal courage to stay present with others when they are looking to the leader for answers that the leader does not have. Yet followers respect leaders who are not afraid to admit that they do not have the answers. They are encouraged when a leader communicates the belief that they will find the answers by working together. This presence during trying times is a tremendous gift the leader gives to others.

When these three elements of trust are present (competence, congruence, and constancy) followers can place credibility in the leader and his or her actions. Kouzes and Posner (1993a, 1993b) have studied credibility extensively. They believe credibility relates to how a leader earns the trust and confidence of his or her constituency. They have found that "people want leaders who hold to an ethic of service and are genuinely respectful of the intelligence and contributions of their constituents. They want leaders who will put principles ahead of politics and other people before self-interests" (1993b, p. xvii). Credibility is a way of maintaining or regaining people's faith in their institutions and the individuals who lead them.

Support. The constancy of support that the leader offers is a vital issue affecting the quality of the leader-follower relationship. To *support* is to nurture or to provide sustenance, a two-way street going from followers to leaders and from leaders to followers. Consistency of support is critical; without it, trust wavers. If a leader offers support only when everything is going smoothly and then withdraws it during vulnerable times, it is of virtually no value because the followers cannot count on it. The net result in the relationship is one of uneasiness, of being uncertain whether this time the support will be there or not. Ironically, followers most need support during the times when leaders most frequently withdraw it—when mistakes occur and when someone makes poor decisions or errors in judgment. In a healthy relationship, the giver freely offers consistent and visible support to the receiver.

A leader's response to mistakes or errors is often the clue followers have as to the consistency of support that the leader extends. If punitive consequences are the norm, people do not feel supported. Punitive consequences to mistakes can occur in the form of shaming, blaming, humiliating followers, or reducing their future opportunities. Simply stepping in and taking over, relieving the follower of responsibility for correcting the consequences that resulted, can appear as a lack of support. Interestingly, if others observe the leader engaging in negative, punitive behavior with any follower, the action is enough to damage trust with followers not even directly involved. This is not to imply that a leader should not take appropriate consequences for a person making the same mistakes repeatedly.

Behavior. Constancy may also refer to stability of personal characteristics. The leader who experiences extreme fluctuations in mood, who is quick to anger, or who responds with knee-jerk reactions may have more trust problems with followers. Take the leader who is excessively positive about ideas, unrealistically optimistic about the chances for a project's success, and effusive with praise on one day but exactly the opposite on the next day. Followers are left with an uncomfortable feeling of uncertainty, which impairs trust. Although it is next to impossible for a leader to be completely balanced and thoroughly predictable, the degree to which the leader avoids these surprises enhances followers' trust in the relationship. Consistency of behavior is important.

Repairing Broken Trust

The three key ingredients of competence, congruence, and constancy must all be present for a healthy relationship. If mistrust is present, examining these three areas can help to sort out the probable causes. When mistrust is apparent in potential followers, one possible approach to the solution is for the leader to ask the followers: What has happened to damage trust? Leaders with the courage to ask this question are often rewarded with insight. Unless the leader asks the question sincerely, however, followers may be reluctant to discuss situations in which they believe a leader let them down. Bennis (1989) points out that good leaders encourage respectful dissent so that they can know the truth about a situation, even if it is not what the leader would like to hear. In fact, good leaders need people around who have contrary views and serve as devil's advocates.

Rogers (1994) identifies three steps to repairing broken trust:

1. Acknowledging
2. Apologizing
3. Making amends

Acknowledging. The first step, acknowledging broken trust, is tough for many leaders. Few leaders purposefully set out to destroy trust, and admitting that something has happened to damage it in this relationship is difficult. In fact, some leaders prefer to call it something else, anything else, rather than accept it as a lack of trust. Some people believe that acknowledging a lack of trust implies a personal fault of some kind, and this belief makes honestly examining these situations especially onerous.

Susan is a senior vice president in a community hospital in Texas. The hierarchy in her organization is very rigid, and rules and policies are plentiful. One expectation is that all employees, including managers and executives, use a time card. For years employees were required to have the individual to whom they reported sign their time cards, but managers and executives did not follow this rule. Problems developed with one manager, including questionable entries and inaccuracies in recording sick or absent time. As a result, Susan began to require that all managers and executives have their time cards signed. The reaction was predictable: people felt they were no longer trusted. Susan was adamant that her requirement for the double check on the time cards was just policy, but her assurances did nothing to assuage their feelings. When pushed, she finally admitted that she wanted to enforce the policy because of performance problems with one individual. Even when confronted directly, she continued to deny that there were any trust issues. It was clearly a lack of trust (albeit well deserved) in the one individual who had been found altering and falsifying time cards.

Apologizing. Apologizing for a breach of trust is difficult for many leaders. This does not mean accepting fault for something that is not the leader's responsibility. If it is the leader's responsibility, the apology may sound like this: "I made a mistake, and I am sorry"; or "I am sorry that my decision has caused these difficulties for you." If the leader is not culpable, the apology may sound different: "I am sorry to hear you feel this way; the decision was right for this situation"; or "I am sorry that is what you heard. Let me try explaining this again." Another possibility is simply to say, "I am sorry that happened."

Apologies are very difficult for some people because they believe that apologizing diminishes their stature or damages the other person's respect for them. Many managers and executives have been socialized in a hierarchical system in which formal leaders just do not admit mistakes to employees, perhaps because they believe it may weaken their authority. The problem with this attitude is that what one most hopes to avoid is exactly what occurs: people lose respect for individuals who cannot admit they were wrong or made a mistake.

In one community hospital undergoing a major work-redesign initiative in the late 1990s, employees showed significant distrust of administration. Five years previously a layoff had occurred, and executives had made several very visible and devastating mistakes in the way they handled the process. While the executives talked about these mistakes behind closed doors, employees talked about them openly. The executives closed ranks and never talked with employees about these mistakes. The pervasive feeling was an antagonistic workforce that did not trust the executives to manage this new challenge because employees did not believe the executives had learned anything from the layoff. How different the environment might have been if the executives and employees held an open dialogue and shared ideas about what they had learned during and since the layoff.

Making Amends. The last step in repairing broken trust is to make amends. If something can be corrected or if a behavior is not repeated, these are ways of making amends. Sometimes the easiest thing to do is to ask, "How can I make this right? How can I make amends?" In many instances, an apology is enough. However, if there is behavior to be changed and one makes the commitment to do so, the leader must follow through on this commitment. Reestablishing trust may take longer than expected. People will be watching closely to determine whether they can believe the leader's promises.

Making amends also implies some reciprocal behavior from the follower. If the leader changes his or her behavior and maintains it, followers at some point need to let go of past wrongs. A leader in one organization found that his early behavior when first appointed to his position resulted in a reputation that still haunts him ten years later! This individual needs to address this lack of trust from followers, and he should perhaps ask for their trust.

Mutual Respect

The second essential element in forming a healthy relationship is mutual respect between leader and follower, which means having esteem for or valuing the other person or his or her skills or characteristics. In a leadership relationship, one can offer respect in two ways. In the first, the leader offers respect unconditionally to followers. This respect is not contingent on superficial attributes such as position, education, or socioeconomic status but recognizes the contributions, both actual and potential, of the individual. Relating to followers as colleagues is a characteristic of a transformational leader (Burns, 1978). This does not mean that you would not respect an individual's achievements in education or position but that you would not withhold respect from an individual because he or she does not have a particular level of education or position of authority.

In health care, because we extend unconditional respect to patients and families regardless of their situation, we often assume that this same respect exists among health care workers. All too often, however, people offer respect merely because of the status or authority inherent in a title. Just as a person leaving a position often becomes a nonentity because that person no longer has a title, management may not recognize certain employees as leaders because these staff have no formal title. Some believe that individuals with particular educational qualifications are most capable or are the only ones with the ability to solve certain problems. These are all examples of respect based on superficial attributes. A leader understands fully that another situation may cause a reversal of positions, placing the leader in a follower position.

The respect a leader extends to followers is a result of a sincere belief that followers are partners, that they have ideas, abilities, solutions, and a keen interest in the situation. Max DePree (1989) says that the excellent leader begins with understanding the diversity and breadth of people's gifts, talents, and skills. "Understanding and accepting diversity enables us to see that each of us is needed. It also enables us to begin to think about being abandoned to the strengths of others, of admitting that we cannot know or do everything" (p. 9). Extending respect to others includes seeking input, soliciting opinions and ideas, and then using these in making decisions. It also means providing freedom within the relationship, allowing a give-and-take to occur.

We may also offer respect based on performance. In other words, we observe a person's skills or abilities and see that he or she obtains desirable outcomes. This type of respect may be differential: we do not guarantee the same level of respect to all people but base it on their individual performance. In this case, we withdraw respect if the individual does not achieve appropriate or desirable outcomes. In other words, the individual who makes repeated mistakes and does not learn from them may experience the consequences of losing others' respect and even being removed from a position.

Communication

The third essential element of healthy relationships is open and honest communication. No leader is effective without the ability to communicate with others. This involves excellent communication skills and a willingness to talk through issues. A leader may be highly skilled but unwilling to do the time-consuming work of communicating. Because of the scope and importance of this element, Chapter Four is devoted entirely to communication skills.

Creating a Trust-Based Organizational Climate

Healthy relationships are the foundation of a trust-based organizational climate. Effective leaders continually scan their environment and the reactions of organizational members to assess levels of trust. We are becoming increasingly aware of the direct correlation between a positive, trust-based work environment and the competitive advantage of the organization. "We are a society in search of trust. The less we find it, the more precious it becomes. An organization in which people earn one another's trust, and that commands trust from the public, has a competitive advantage. It can draw the best people, inspire customer loyalty, reach out successfully to new markets, and provide more innovative products and services" (Ciancutti and Steding, 2001, p. ix).

This message echoes the earlier work of Reina and Reina (1999), who examined closely the issues of trust and betrayal in today's workplaces. They write that "Unmet expectations, disappointments, broken trust, and betrayals aren't restricted to big events like restructurings and downsizings. They crop up every day on the job. Leaders are beginning to realize that people's trust and commitment to the organization affect their performance" (p. ix). Reina and Reina offer a model for understanding the complex and emotional issue of trust and betrayal in today's organization. They believe it is possible to create an organizational climate in which transformative trust exists. Four core characteristics that produce transformative trust are conviction, courage, compassion, and community.

In the book *Built on Trust* (2001), Ciancutti and Steding talk about intentionally creating trust in the organization. They offer a model for deliberately and systematically establishing and maintaining high levels of trust. The steps include the following:

Closure with all communication. This means coming to a specific agreement about who will do what and by when.

Commitment, which is a positive intention to complete what the parties agreed to with no conditions. If one is unable to follow through or fulfill the commitment as agreed to for any reason, then one speaks up immediately.

Communication is direct, open, and honest, which eliminates dysfunctional forms such as talking behind people's backs, withholding information, taking part in hallway conversations, and so on.

Speedy resolution, which refers to clearing up unresolved issues as soon as they become apparent and as soon as possible.

Respect, using tact and respect in communications.

Responsibility, which refers to the concept that each person owns his or her own problems but remains willing and able to give the other help.

In addition to these steps, Ciancutti and Steding (2001) include discussion of other principles such as being responsive to each other, telling the truth, agreeing to a no-surprise practice, handling issues at the lowest possible level in the organization, and relying on managers who serve as daily role models in each of these aspects.

Leadership Relationships in the Future

Establishing and cultivating a healthy relationship with followers is an initial step in developing the ability to influence others. This can be accomplished by ensuring that the three elements of a healthy relationship—trust, mutual respect, and communication—are in place. Understanding the concepts of collaboration and partnership is also important because these describe the nature of today's effective leader-follower relationship.

Collaboration and *partnering* are terms similar in meaning. *Collaboration* refers to work or labor accomplished together, and *partner* is derived from the word *partake*, meaning "to share." The essence of a successful leader's relationship with followers and key stakeholders is a combination of collaboration and partnership. *Collaboration* became a buzzword in the 1990s, found in many journal articles and workshop titles. But like most buzzwords, it is one that people overuse and misuse without a true understanding of the concept. A good leader may not need to know the actual definition but certainly needs to live the concept in relation with followers and colleagues.

Collaboration

Collaboration has multiple meanings, but the most useful is that of working together, especially in a joint intellectual effort. In leader-follower collaboration, it means interactions between leader and follower that enable the knowledge and skills of both to synergistically influence the decision the two are making or the work they are accomplishing (Manion, 1989). *Synergy* is a biochemical term meaning that the whole is greater than the sum of its parts. In the leadership context, it means that when the leader and follower work together, they are likely to generate more and better solutions and alternatives than either would by working alone. Dictionary definitions rarely bring a concept fully to life. To more completely understand collaboration, examining the relationship between coordination, cooperation, and sharing mutual work is helpful (Baggs and Schmitt, 1988). These three ingredients compose the whole of collaboration.

Coordination

Coordination is the summary of individual ideas. It occurs when two or more people come together and share their points of view and experiences to ensure a harmonious combination or interaction. One executive team meets regularly on Monday mornings for a short time, sharing plans for the week, discussing major issues, and briefly reviewing its members' calendars. Their intent is to coordinate efforts. Another example is a patient-care conference in a patient-care department that is often held for a similar purpose. The individuals from the different disciplines or shifts come together to compare their assessments of patients and to coordinate their efforts. Coordination is based on sharing information.

Cooperation

Cooperation implies planning and working together in an actively helpful manner, more than being passively cooperative or simply accommodating. Cooperation as it relates to collaboration means meeting the other person's needs yet being assertive in meeting one's own needs; being assertive and uncooperative, on the other hand, is being competitive.

Sharing Mutual Work

Sharing mutual work in collaboration means sharing goals, planning, problem solving, decision making, and responsibility. Contrast this with consultation, in which sharing occurs during the planning phase but allows the individual to proceed alone in implementation.

True collaboration requires all three elements in healthy amounts: coordination, cooperation, and mutual work. Too often a leader makes a decision and then expects others to coordinate and cooperate in its implementation. The leader may honestly feel that he or she is being collaborative because there is a general feeling of cooperation. However, unless both parties made the decision mutually, it is not collaboration in the true sense of the word. The very basis of any partnering relationship is collaboration.

Partnership

Successful relationships of the future will be characterized as partnerships, which are forming at all levels in our society. Communities are forming partnerships with businesses and industries. Former competitors, such as Apple and IBM, are creating business partnerships. In a community in the Midwest, two hospitals of competing systems are considering building together a third facility needed in their area. Strategic partnerships are appearing with more regularity in health care, between health care systems as well as individual organizations (Blouin and Brent, 1997). Managerial partnerships are found at the executive and managerial level (Manion, Sieg, and Watson, 1998; Heenan and Bennis, 1999). Tomorrow's leader needs to work in partnership with others. It is the very essence of the leader-follower relationship. As Heenan and Bennis (p. 5) write: "In a world of increasing interdependence and ceaseless technological change, even the greatest of Great Men or Women simply can't get the job done alone. As a result, we need to rethink our most basic concepts of leadership."

The philosophy and approach of "every man for himself" in organization life is gradually going by the wayside. In the past, organizations often rewarded managers for the size of their turf. The larger their budget and the more direct reports and greater number of personnel in their departments, the greater their status. Organization environments were competitive and predominantly unhealthy. If the organization was to meet one manager's request, it would deny another's. Today the manager who is a leader understands the importance of forming alliances and partnering with colleagues to accomplish results. The effective leader of tomorrow will be one who is able to form collaborative associations with others to achieve the organization's mission. This is much more complex than it first appears because an individual, group, or organization may at one time be a competitor, a partner, a distributor, or a supplier. Balancing these complex relationships takes a high level of maturity.

Although successful leaders will be those who are able and willing to be partners to others, the task is not as easy as it may seem, because not everyone is suited to being a partner. Partnering may well be the highest level of interpersonal development. Stephen Covey, author of *The Seven Habits of Highly Effective People* (1989), identifies stages of development and their ramifications in the professional world. As individuals develop, they progress from a state of dependence to independence and then to interdependence. Each of these stages of development represents significant and substantial progress. In the stage of dependence, the individual relies on others. In the stage of independence, there is more reliance on the self; the individual has taken responsibility for behavior and ownership of feelings and accomplishments. At this point, the individual is capable of moving to the higher interdependence level of development to work effectively with others and share responsibility and recognition.

Interdependence

Covey (1989) points out that only independent people can make the choice to become interdependent. So highly dependent people have difficulty moving into true interdependence. Independent people may choose not to become interdependent and in fact may see relinquishing control to others or sharing decision making as a weakness. Executives in health care systems across the country are learning to balance the mixture of independence and interdependence as they partner with colleagues to lead in a variety of ways.

This development continuum, as illustrated in Figure 2.2, is significant to understanding the leadership relationship. Both Bennis (1989) and DePree (1989) describe leaders as seasoned, mature people who have recognized the need for—and have consciously chosen—interdependence with their followers. The excellent leader does not go it alone but derives energy and ideas from follower-colleagues. In a healthy leader-follower relationship, there is true synergy: the two achieve more together than either could achieve alone. Neither leader nor follower exists in a vacuum; they function in a reciprocal relationship.

Interestingly, the concept of partnership has been with us since the earliest of times. In *The Chalice and the Blade*, Eisler (1987) describes the shift from a partnership societal model in the earliest

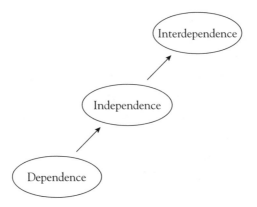

Figure 2.2. The Development Continuum

human history to a dominator model. It is clear from her research that "war and the 'war of the sexes' are neither divinely nor biologically ordained" (p. xv). Based on her understanding and interpretation of historical artifacts and findings, the earliest human societies existed in which "difference is not necessarily equated with inferiority or superiority" (p. xvii) and neither gender is subjugated to the other. The application of this in today's organizations is clear. Many people are involved in organizations that are "working to create more mutual relationships, democratic institutions, and equitable societies. . . . they want personal and social power to be used with and for others, not over or against them. They believe that conflict can be resolved collaboratively and peacefully" (Eisler and Loye, 1998, p. viii).

Collective Responsibility and Accountability

In any partnership, the members must retain a sense of personal responsibility and accountability. But a new dimension is added in the leader-follower relationship: the sharing of collective responsibility and accountability. For the relationship to thrive and continue to flourish, all elements of a healthy relationship discussed in this chapter must exist on both sides of the partnering agreement. The leader must be trustworthy, as must be the followers. Respect is mutual and communication two-way. Without these things, the partnership withers and dies.

Conclusion

The quality of the leader-follower relationship directly correlates to the effectiveness of the leader and ability of all to achieve necessary outcomes. Emotional intelligence and a relationship based on trust and confidence, mutual respect, and honest communication create a vital association. The nature of the relationship is one of collaboration and partnership—neither of which is easy to attain but is worth every ounce of effort it takes. Relationships in today's world are "parallel and simultaneous, connected, murky, multiple, and interdependent" (Bennis, 1989, p. 101). Forming healthy relationships is complex, ever changing, and always challenging for the exemplary leader.

Conversation Points

1. Use the three essential ingredients of a healthy relationship presented here (trust, respect, and communication) to assess the quality of your work relationships.

2. Are there issues of trust between people in your department? In your organization?

3. As a leader, what actions demonstrate your trust of other people?

4. Think of a time you felt betrayed by someone or something that happened in your workplace. How did you handle it? Do you carry the sense of betrayal with you, or were you able to resolve it?

Building Commitment

Getting Others to Follow

Compliance is a matter of the mind;
commitment engages the heart.

Jo Manion, From Management to Leadership

L eadership is more than influencing others to follow a specific
direction; it is creating a desire in the followers to do so. With
a healthy leader-follower relationship, followers are more likely to
choose the path the leader indicates. A healthy relationship, however, is only the beginning. The leader will be more effective if he
or she differentiates the concepts of personal and organizational
commitment and also understands the difference between commitment and compliance. Leaders who understand the various forms
of organizational commitment as well as the stages of commitment
formation and key factors that result in commitment can consciously choose behaviors to support this process. With the current
emphasis on finding effective employee-retention strategies, understanding the basis of personal and organizational commitment
is needed to avoid unnecessary frustration and the expense of the

Note: This chapter is adapted from Jo Manion, "Strengthening Organizational
Commitment" in *The Health Care Manager,* © 2004. Used by permission of the
publisher: Lippincott Williams & Wilkins, Baltimore, Md.

shotgun approach, in which we try everything in the hopes that something works.

Although teaching people how to build commitment through reading and classroom work is difficult, if not impossible, a thorough understanding of the concept reveals several specific steps that leaders can take to increase followers' level of commitment. Peter Senge (1996, p. 10) describes the importance of commitment that leaders and followers share when he writes about leading learning organizations: "We have seen no examples where significant progress has been made without leadership from local line managers, and many examples where sincerely committed CEOs have failed to generate any significant momentum." In other words, no leader accomplishes a major change or program initiative alone; it requires a vital partnership with followers, all working in concert to carry out the plan.

Compliance

In the past, when formal managers were considered the primary source of leadership in the organization and the old command-and-control methodology was still acceptable, compliance seemed fairly easy to attain. Followers were simply told what to do, and they were expected to conform or acquiesce regardless of their own opinions or ideas. Two factors today make mere compliance inadequate. The first is the nature of the workforce. A clear majority of the members of today's health care organizations are older, more mature and experienced; and they feel more involved in their work than ever. Second, the changes occurring are no longer mere tweaks to the system but are instead fundamental, complex alterations to the very way we deliver service. The success of this deep level of change requires more than mere compliance on the part of those individuals who will implement these changes. Compliance means conformance. People do what they have been directed or asked to do. There may be very little personal involvement. Commitment is a personal pledge to a position or issue. It is a matter of giving one-self in trust to the issue or solution. Compliance is a matter of the mind; commitment engages the heart.

Commitment

Understanding the underpinnings of personal and organizational commitment is crucial for health care leaders in today's business en-vironment. Accelerating change, increasing organizational chal-lenges and crises, workforce shortages, and mounting environmental pressures make the need for committed and fully engaged employ-ees more important than ever.

The Concept

Commitment is the act of pledging or engaging oneself. To commit is to bind or obligate oneself, as in committing to a promise, a cer-tain course of action, or even another person. A review of the clas-sic organization development literature sheds further light on the concept. Brickman and his colleagues (Brickman, Wortman, and Sorrentino, 1987, p. 2) studied commitment extensively and say it is "a force that stabilizes individual behavior under circumstances where the individual would otherwise be tempted to change that behavior. . . . Commitment is whatever it is that makes a person engage or continue in a course of action when difficulties or posi-tive alternatives influence the person to abandon the effort."

We see commitment in the workplace daily when people remain at work despite unpleasant or rapidly deteriorating conditions. All of us can remember days when everything seemed to go wrong and we would rather have been somewhere, anywhere, else. It was our commitment that kept us at work.

The early work of Rosabeth Moss Kanter (1972) included a study of thirty U.S. utopian communities to determine whether their com-mitment practices were related to their chances of success. Contrary to a prevalent notion at the time that utopian communities exist for people who want the freedom to do their own thing, Kanter found a general tendency for the most stable and successful communes to spend more time and effort instilling commitment in their members. In other words, they made an effort to ensure that their members acted in ways beneficial to the community.

Commitment contains a directional element (Trigg, 1973). An individual can never be just committed; one must be committed to something or someone. Commitments are not free-floating but instead are attached to a person or a thing. Commitment also implies a strong evaluative element: people must believe in the truth and inherent value of that to which they commit. Commitment indicates a belief that an organization or job is a good one, worth supporting, and important in some way. People do not commit to organizations that they believe are trivial, deceitful, or potentially corrupt. They make a judgment about an organization or job in light of their values.

Presupposing certain beliefs, commitment involves a personal dedication to the actions those beliefs imply. So commitment is more than belief; it is a strong enough belief that actually *compels* action. To illustrate this observation, consider the example of membership in a professional association. Members obviously evidence differing levels of commitment. One may believe that the association advances the profession, which is of value, but may choose not to join and support the association. There is no action, thus no commitment, even though the individual may recognize the association's value. Or one may join and pay dues but not participate in committees, task forces, or local membership meetings. One's actions show some commitment to the association. On the other hand, one may be an active member of the association, involved and participating, contributing in numerous ways. This shows a higher level of commitment.

The essence of commitment is in the "relationship between the 'want to' and 'have to.' . . . Commitment involves three elements: a positive element, a negative element, and a bond between the two" (Brickman, Wortman, and Sorrentino, 1987, p. 6). This makes commitment a distinctive and compelling psychological process. The connection between the two elements, not merely their joint presence, is critical for commitment. Furthermore, the nature of this connection and bonding determines the nature of the commitment.

Even the most absorbing of commitments has negative elements. Examples include the spouse who nurses a partner through a devastating and lengthy terminal illness; the manager who spends inordinate amounts of time at work, often at the expense of personal relationships; the highly skilled surgeon who has made heavy sacrifices to learn those skills and runs risks daily in exercising these skills. And even the most alienated commitment contains a positive element. "People who stay with a job or marriage after the life has gone out of it may no longer have the reason that initially drew them, but they still have reasons, they still have something of value that they do not wish to lose. . . . Thus the pension the person derives from the job, or the reputation and security from the marriage, become more valuable" (Brickman, Wortman, and Sorrentino, 1987, p. 7). In other words, the investment the individual made in the commitment has become more important than the original reason for the commitment.

> People experience commitment in at least two different ways. If the negative element is salient, persistence is the manifestation. If the positive element is stronger, enthusiasm is manifest. Persistence characterizes behavior that people continue to enact despite their sense that it calls for them to make sacrifices and resist temptations—they may have to work hard and resist the pleasure of quitting. Enthusiasm characterizes behavior that people enact without ambivalence about what the behavior costs, out of a sense that the behavior itself is meaningful. Persistence in commitment reflects the call of duty; enthusiasm goes beyond the call of duty. (Brickman, Wortman, and Sorrentino, 1987, p. 10)

This is an important cue for leaders in the workplace. If people seem to have lost their enthusiasm, this does not necessarily mean that they will leave the organization; but it may mean that the negative aspects of the job have overtaken the positive. Logically, when persistence is all that is keeping the person in the job, the individual is likely closer to the next step, severing the commitment.

Interestingly, adversity plays an important role in the formation of commitment (Lydon and Zanna, 1990). Without the negative element or adversity and the existence of alternatives that the individual must sacrifice, that person has not made a true choice. Adversity can serve as a catalyst in the development of commitment. It can strengthen and affirm a commitment. Researchers have most commonly studied this in the realm of romantic commitment, finding that romantic love develops more strongly in the face of opposition. This chapter will address ramifications in the workplace more fully in another section.

Stages of Commitment

Commitment has five stages, and these help us understand the process and issues related to each stage (Brickman, Wortman, and Sorrentino, 1987). Briefly described here, these stages also give insight into the breaking as well as the making of commitments.

Stage One

Commitments in stage one are *exploratory*. During this stage we explore a potential activity or relationship with concern only for the positive elements that might make further exploration worthwhile. These are precommitments because they often involve a positive orientation toward the potential object of commitment and significant reflection has not yet occurred. Beginning commitments are often positive and somewhat superficial. Recall your early stages of a job search or your exploration of a possible promotion.

Stage Two

Commitments in stage two can be best described as *testing*. By this point, one has encountered some negative elements or events, and one assesses the willingness and ability to accommodate these. We may have been involved in testing the environment, for example, to determine the manager or coworker's willingness to make concessions and contribute in some meaningful way to the employment relationship. Or we test ourselves to determine our ability to solve the problem or accomplish a task or activity. This stage also involves a search for information, but the focus is on negative and troubling aspects rather than the positive attributes inherent in stage one. The focus at this point is external, and the crisis is one of encountering unfamiliar and perhaps unexpected events. We discover that the honeymoon is over. The new job or organization has failed in some way to meet our expectations.

Stage Three

Passionate describes the commitments of stage three. This stage is characterized by the first major synthesis of positive and negative elements as well as recognition of the entire process as a commitment. Commitments of this stage are fiercely positive, with denial of any negative features; and such commitments are highly self-conscious (Brickman, Wortman, and Sorrentino, 1987). The individual at this stage is sometimes fanatical, acting in ways that are rigid and without regard to costs. It is almost as if we need a more rigid, positive view in order to remain committed once we have a more realistic view of negative elements in the situation.

Stage Four

The commitments of stage four are *quiet*. This stage emerges more slowly as the energy we need to maintain the passion of stage three fades along with the ambiguity of the previous stage. This leads to the crisis of this stage, which occurs because we have attained the object of the commitment and now must focus energy on retaining and sustaining the commitment. Familiarity and comfort, characteristic of this stage, can undermine the effort required to sustain it. As Maxwell says, "Commitment is the will of the mind to finish what the heart has begun long after the emotion in which the promise was made has passed" (Maxwell, 2003, p. 8).

The orientation of this stage is intrinsic, with the threat coming from inside the person. Boredom is the crisis. Many who reach this stage in their work commitments begin looking around within the job at this time, seeking new opportunities or new ways to experience challenge again.

Stage Five

Stage-five commitments are *integral.* These commitments represent a higher level of integration of both positive and negative elements, with the integration being more flexible and complex than earlier bonding. The structure that exists allows awareness of both the positive and negative elements or the entire commitment to flow in and out of consciousness. During stage five, "individuals have the capacity to treat their commitments in a cognitively simple or mindless way, simply acting out of habit or following a well-known script" (Brickman, Wortman, and Sorrentino, 1987, p. 179).

These five stages are helpful for understanding how we establish commitments and the process we go through when making commitments. They provide increased clarity about the reactions we can expect, and this can be reassuring for people who may be feeling confused by the differing dynamics of the various stages.

Perhaps one of the most important reasons to understand the stages of forming a commitment is because such understanding increases our appreciation that forming a commitment is a *process.* As such, commitments are dynamic rather than static, changing in their characteristics as they become deeper and more strongly affirmed.

Organizational Commitment

Researchers have studied commitment in a myriad of different contexts, but the focus here is commitment in the work setting. There are many definitions of organizational commitment, with the simplest being an employee's expressed intent to stay. Wiener (1982) points out that behaviors resulting in organizational commitment possess the following characteristics: (1) they reflect some personal sacrifice made for the sake of the organization; (2) they show persistence; and (3) the commitments indicate a personal preoccupation with the organization, such as devoting a great deal of time to organization-related activities. These characteristics vary in degree depending on the strength of the commitment.

Other elements of organizational commitment that scholars have identified include a strong belief and acceptance of the organization's goals, a willingness to exert effort on the organization's behalf, a strong desire to maintain membership in the organization, and group cohesiveness (Kanter, 1972; Makin, Cooper, and Cox, 1996). Group cohesiveness is the "ability of people to 'stick together,' to develop the mutual attraction and collective strength to withstand threats to the group's existence" (Kanter, 1972, p. 67).

Types of Organizational Commitment

Extensive research has revealed at least three specific types of organizational commitment. Understanding these enables leaders to influence the level of employees' commitment more significantly.

Continuance Commitment

This form of commitment is based on the fact that the employee recognizes the benefits to be gained for aligning with the system as well as sacrifices to be made or costs to be paid. This is a cognitive process. The balance between costs and rewards must tip in the direction of rewards in order for an employee to remain in the system. Early research on commitment focused on side bets (Becker, 1960).

In the organizational context of employment, the term *side bet* can refer to anything of value that the individual has invested, including money, ego, time, and effort that the employee would lose or might deem worthless if he or she were to leave the organization. Such investments might include contributions to nonvested pension plans, the development of organization-specific skills or status, or any specific organizational benefits that no other organization can duplicate. Thus, the threat of a loss binds the person to the organization.

Employees committed to the organization primarily for financial reasons such as pay and benefits are not as likely to be committed to the organization's values (Mayer and Schoorman, 1998). In fact, they may actually become a liability to the organization because of higher than normal levels of dissatisfaction and lower levels of job performance (Meyer and others, 1989).

Affective Commitment

Affective commitment occurs as a result of events and occurrences that increase an emotional connection with the employee's work group and lead to increased group cohesiveness (Kanter, 1972; Iverson and Buttigieg, 1999). Over the years we have seen that lower rates of turnover have been related to strong emotional and affiliative ties with the work group. When the commitment to relationships within the workplace is strong, the ties of emotion bind group members to each other as well as to the community they form. Today a sense of community within the workplace has become increasingly important for many people because it may be the only source of community in which they participate. Decreasing involvement in family, religious institutions, and neighborhood activities; increased geographical distances from family members and childhood communities; and extremely harried and full work lives have all combined to escalate a general feeling of isolation and disconnectedness from the typical communities of the past (Manion and Bartholomew, 2004).

Affective commitment is based on the strength of positive feelings that increase the emotional bond. It also explains why turnover is more costly than simply its monetary impact. Turnover ruptures relationships and threatens the work group's cohesiveness (Barney, 2002; Manion, 2000a; Manion, 2000b; Manion, 2004a).

Normative Commitment

The final form of organizational commitment comes from the recognition that one's personal values and beliefs fit with the organization. "Commitment to uphold norms, obey the authority of the group, and support its values, involves primarily a person's evaluative orientations. When demands made by the system are evaluated as right, moral, just, or expressing one's own values, obedience to these demands is regarded as appropriate" (Makin, Cooper, and Cox, 1996, p. 69). This is known as moral commitment or *normative commitment*, and there is less deviance and challenge to authority when it exists.

This explains at least partially why congruence between an organization and a leader's stated values and behavior is so critical. A breach in moral commitment occurs when employees perceive the organization or leader acting in ways inconsistent with stated beliefs or in ways significantly different from the employee's values. We have all seen the effects of this at one time or other. For example, one midsize community hospital in the Midwest states clearly that its most important value is quality patient care. Yet employees openly and disdainfully argue that the organization's true value is quality *physician* care, because in numerous and highly visible examples over the years, executive behavior has not supported the organization's slogan "patients first." Instead, what the physician wants rather than what the patient needs has guided decisions and action. What started as a catchy phrase meant to exemplify the organization's values has become a liability in building employee commitment.

Although these different types of commitments may lead to stronger organizational support and affiliation, the nature of each of these links to employees is quite different. "Employees with a strong affective commitment remain with the organization because they want to, whereas those with strong continuance commitment remain because they need to" (Meyer and Allen, 1984, p. 152). As a result, the daily performance and behavior of these employees are different. Those who value and want to remain part of the organization are likely to exert considerable effort on the organization's behalf, whereas those who feel compelled to stay to avoid financial or other costs may do little more than the minimum required to retain their employment.

Today's health care organization contains many employees who "stayed but left" or who "psychologically resigned" a long time before. Coworkers can easily identify these people because they rarely behave in a manner that exhibits any affective commitment. In fact, studies have found that employees with continuance commitment evidenced lower job performance and less promotability (Meyer and Allen, 1984). More recent research has found that affective and normative commitment led to positive organizational outcomes (such as lower absenteeism and intention to leave as well as a higher acceptance of change), whereas continuance commitment led to greater inflexibility. In terms of rewards and benefits, merely introducing higher wages increases the person's "perception of low alternatives but has no effect on improving the alignment of employee goals with the organization" (Iverson and Buttigieg, 1999, p. 327).

Leadership Interventions

When a leader understands the essential differences between the three types of organizational commitment, it becomes clear that efforts focusing on strengthening affective and normative commitment bring more long-term benefit. Makin and his colleagues (Makin, Cooper, and Cox, 1996, p. 81) sum it up nicely: "In simple terms . . . people stay with the organization because they *want* to (affective), because they *need* to (continuance), or because they feel they *ought* to (normative)." The more a leader understands about the process of commitment, the more consciously he or she can select leadership behavior that encourages employees to form a commitment. Recognizing the commitments and understanding the dynamics involved in severing or dissolving commitments is also crucial. Otherwise, actions can inadvertently lead employees to further psychological disengagement from the organization. For example, dissolving a team, ending a service, or closing a department may be a wise business decision; but if the organization does not provide emotional support to employees in a way that recognizes the value of their commitment and helps them through this transition, their attachment to the organization as a whole may suffer irreparably.

Organizations most often emphasize continuance commitment during times of workforce shortages, using strategies such as adding recruitment incentives, increasing salaries, and improving benefits. Yet this form of commitment is the weakest and can actually be harmful. Organizations can more likely attain positive outcomes by focusing on and strengthening affective and normative commitment. These two types of commitment are closely related and more likely to develop personal *and* organizational commitment.

Approaches for Building Affective Commitment

How can the leader strengthen affective commitment? This type of commitment is based on the emotional and social connections the employee has with and within the organization. Studies have shown that a person's experiences during the initial months of employment are perhaps the most crucial in developing affective commitment. Focusing efforts to ensure that the organization meets the employee's expectations of it is important. During times of tumultuous change, such as the early days of an employee's employment, there is a need to continually clarify roles and pay attention to the formation of healthy relationships with new employees.

The nature and quality of an employee's work experience during his or her tenure in an organization influences commitment.

The work experience is a major socializing force, and it significantly influences the extent to which employees form affective attachments with the organization. Experiences found to influence commitment included the work group's attitudes toward the organization, organizational dependability and trust, and perception of one's importance. Additionally, efforts that support the development of healthy working relationships in work groups are a crucial beginning for the formation of this strong commitment. Peer relationships are important, but so is the relationship of the individual with organizational leaders and others with whom interaction is common (such as patients and families, people in other departments, and physicians). Healthy relationships, as discussed in Chapter Two, are based on trust, mutual respect, and open communication.

Approaches for Building Normative Commitment

There are three essential components to building normative commitment, as shown in Figure 3.1:

- Shared values

- A common mission or purpose

- A shared vision

Identifying and working from shared values, a common sense of mission, and a mutually developed and held clear vision are three concrete ways a leader builds normative commitment among followers. The more fully these exist and the degree to which each has meaning for the followers, the greater the level of commitment. In recent years each of these concepts has become a buzzword.

These concepts, though simple in meaning, are rarely easy to attain. Implied in each is that the leader first has extraordinary insight into what is personally and organizationally important in his or her leadership practice and can comfortably and clearly articulate it to others. Then the concept is more likely to become personally rele-

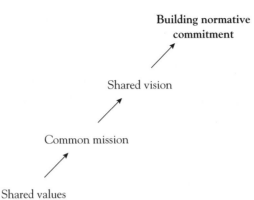

Figure. 3.1. Steps for Building Normative Commitment

vant to the followers, who deem it important enough to commit wholeheartedly to the effort and help the group attain results.

Deeply held values, a clear sense of mission, and a shared vision are often leadership attributes rather than specific skills. Guided classroom activities may help a leader clarify his or her beliefs in each area but cannot develop them if they are not already present. Usually forged by life's experiences and the development of one's personality and beliefs, these elements reveal themselves over time. For optimum leadership effectiveness, these are not only present but are vibrant and vital within the leader's day-to-day practice.

Shared Values

Essential to developing commitment is the presence of shared values between leaders and followers and between individuals and the organization. Values are pervasive, deep-seated standards that affect all aspects of life. They are beliefs that one holds to be of worth, such as the value of kindness, freedom, or teamwork. There are group and individual values, all of which may exist simultaneously for a person. Societal values are beliefs that most members of a society hold, such as independence, personal freedom, and choice. Organization values are beliefs common to most people in an establishment, such as service to others, competence, and quality. Family values, although sometimes construed as a political statement in today's world, are simply beliefs about what's important within the family unit (however it is defined), such as commitment, support, honoring each other, and caring. Personal values are beliefs that the individual holds, such as integrity, honesty, challenge, and achievement. In addition to these categories, an individual may hold work values; in the case of a leader, these become the person's leadership values. These are the beliefs they hold for this aspect of their lives. Respect for others, integrity, honesty, and competence are examples of what a leader's values might be.

Aligned Values

In an individual who experiences a high level of congruence among the different aspects of his or her life, these values overlap and are in sync with one another. High levels of energy and enthusiasm for life are the result. Each arena of life supports and reinforces the others. Personal power and effectiveness are at a peak. Contradiction among values in these different areas creates dissonance, resulting in disturbance for an individual. Three choices exist at this point. The individual may take steps to reduce the dissonance, perhaps by redefining the value to make it fit the situation. Another option is to suppress the uncomfortable and possibly painful feelings that arise and deny that there is any discomfort. This happens when we turn away and pretend not to see a situation that offends one of our values. The third alternative for a person of integrity is to take steps to change that aspect of life that holds unacceptable contradictions in values. We can do this by addressing and bringing forth concerns about the situation or even removing ourselves from the dissonant situation permanently.

Prioritizing Values

Life is about choices. An individual with integrity is continually aware of the values that serve as a foundation for his or her life and recognizes the choices that must be made. However, we do not always see or experience choices with great clarity. In any of the arenas of society, organization, family, or work, our stated values may not correspond to the values we truly hold. Rhetoric can easily drown out the truth. A society may say and believe it values personal independence but then inadvertently institute policies and programs that encourage dependence among some citizens. A health care organization may say that it values service and community when in truth its primary focus is on the bottom line, profits, and reputation. The earlier example of one organization's slogan of "patients first" became a source of great dissonance and dissatisfaction for employees as they observed decision after decision that clearly valued physicians first. The credibility gap grew wider with each new decision and subsequent assurance of "patients first." Examining one's feelings of discomfort takes courage, for intuition may be the only thing that is saying something is wrong. An individual with much invested in the current system may find it difficult to admit that their values are not in alignment.

A person of integrity acts in accordance with his or her beliefs. If the values of the organization or group do not match, the individual first assesses the situation to determine whether change is possible. Action follows, based on a belief and hope that the individual can influence the situation. Perhaps leaders in the organization haven't recognized the incongruent messages their decisions are sending. Honest feedback and open dialogue about a perceived mismatch between a stated value and observed behavior need to occur. If nothing changes, the individual's choice becomes clear: stay or leave. "In the work setting, a lack of congruency between personal and organizational values decreases job satisfaction and work productivity and ultimately may lead to job burnout and turnover" (McNeese-Smith and Crook, 2003, p. 260).

In some instances, an individual's assessment of the situation results in a decision to stay so that the individual may meet another highly held personal value. For example, individuals who highly value security and providing for their family's needs may choose to

remain in an organization even though other values are not congruent. Such an individual may hope that this is a temporary situation,
and it is healthier if the individual is able to see clearly the choice
that he or she has made. Too many times an individual remains in a
dissonant situation and suppresses feelings of rebellion against the
differing values. Over the long term, one may even lose sight of or
change one's values, telling oneself that these values are not worth
leaving for.

Courage to choose a different path can be just as difficult when
the conflict is between beneficial values. Which is most important?
Which choice will be most true to the beliefs that the individual
holds dear? Jane, a leader in a health care agency, discovered the
difficulty inherent in choosing between two seemingly good values.
She strongly valued security and stability and had spent most of her
professional career in positions that met these values. Fortunately,
these positions also provided her opportunities to meet other values that she held dear—challenge and achievement. In fact, these
differing values were very compatible for most of her years in health
care. With every challenge she met, every goal she achieved, the
higher rewards and greater financial security and sense of stability
she attained. As a vice president at the corporate level in a home
health agency, she most enjoyed the new projects and service development aspect of her work.

But the company appointed a new CEO, and within six months
Jane became aware that the company's philosophy had changed significantly. Her position became responsible for monitoring and ensuring regulatory compliance and advocating with state legislators.
Although Jane was highly skilled in these areas, she now missed the
challenge and sense of achievement she had previously enjoyed. She
tried to negotiate a role change so that she would be challenged and
excited about work again but was unsuccessful. To make matters
more difficult, the new CEO significantly increased her salary, and
Jane's sense of security was stronger than ever. Her choice was difficult: Would she stay and be true to her value of security and stability,

or would she seek another position full of challenge and the opportunity to grow again? After much soul-searching, she resigned and became an entrepreneur, starting her own business, which over the years became more successful than she dreamed possible. Challenge and achievement were more important than security and stability.

Jane's story illustrates the importance of our values. They guide daily decision making and give a sense of direction in day-to-day existence. Holding the values of security and achievement simultaneously can lead to a crisis point in a career when situations force an individual to choose between remaining in a seemingly secure, well-paying job and seeking a new job with greater challenge. When actions are in accordance with the values one holds, events flow more smoothly.

The Result of Shared Values

When people share values, the result is a tremendous feeling of connection and synergy. Of course, this requires that leaders and followers can clearly define their values. They know what beliefs are most important in their lives. However, if they never discussed their values, anyone may make a false assumption—either that values are in agreement or that they differ. Open dialogue about their beliefs benefits both leaders and followers, because when people share values, they feel united.

The ramifications for a leader who is trying to build commitment to a certain idea are clear. The leader must be absolutely sure about his or her values and how this decision supports these values. If there is incongruity, the leader experiences feelings of dissonance that he or she reflects in subtle ways to followers. When the path chosen is consistent with the leader's values and followers share them, commitment blossoms. The ability to articulate and communicate clearly is critical for this process to succeed. Not only are the technical skills of communication important, the leader also needs the courage to speak from the heart and share his or her deeply held beliefs regardless of the feelings of vulnerability this may create. "The challenge we all face is to find ways to use the workplace as a forum in which to express and embody our deepest values. We can derive a sense of purpose, for example, from mentoring others, or being part of a cohesive team, or simply from a commitment to treating others with respect and care and from communicating positive energy. The real measure of our lives may ultimately be in the small choices we make in each and every moment" (Loehr and Schwartz, 2003, p. 140).

Mission

"The first responsibility of the leader is to define reality" (DePree, 1989, p. 11). In an organizational context, leaders have the task and responsibility of determining both the purpose and the future of their organizations. Beckhard and Pritchard (1992) note that the white-knuckle turbulence of rapid change is forcing most leaders to reexamine the very essence of the organization along with its basic purpose; its identity; and its relationships with customers (internal and external), competitors, and all other key stakeholders. Mycek (1998, p. 26) asks: "What is the true business of healthcare? Is it the 'high-tech, high-touch' blend of dedicated caregivers and state-of-the-art technology that was prophesied in the late 1980s? Or is healthcare purely a commodity—products and services that are bought and sold at the lowest price, on the spot market?" The questions today are becoming more and more difficult. In addition to defining the organization's mission, leaders also need a clear sense of their own mission or purpose.

Strong leaders have a clear sense of mission; they know why they are here and are clear about their purpose. Mission is a reason for existence—of the individual, the project, the team, or the organization. A clear mission defines the purpose and gives direction and focus. It enables an individual to decline opportunities that detract from this true purpose. "It's easy to say 'no' when there is a deeper 'yes' burning inside" (Covey, Merrill, and Merrill, 1994, p. 103).

Over time a person's mission in life evolves. A person grows into a leadership role by fully experiencing life and learning from its many lessons through extensive reading, dialogue with others, travel, trial and error, and observation. People in leadership roles are continual learners, always seeking the lesson in a situation, even when it is difficult or painful. Reflective practice is growing in popularity today (Taylor, 2004). Reflection is a powerful tool that the individual can use to better understand what motivated actions and behaviors, what reactions came of certain situations, how outcomes were attained, and what is really important.

Leadership Mission Statement

Every leader needs a personal mission statement. An individual's mission statement may or may not include a leadership mission statement. For some people, these are two different but compatible statements. A leader needs to distinguish between his or her purpose as an individual and as a leader. One cannot write these statements in only an hour or two. Instead it takes "deep introspection, careful analysis, thoughtful expression, and often many rewrites to produce it in final form" (Covey, 1989, p. 129). It means sorting through a great deal of extraneous material to reach the core reason for one's existence and the way one is to achieve that purpose. The leadership mission statement usually includes the leader's values and often the means by which he or she will achieve the mission.

A strong sense of connection between leaders and followers results from leaders being open and sharing their personal or leadership mission statements. They may initially feel vulnerable and embarrassed because this is a very personal statement. If the leaders are sincere and humble, rather than arrogant and egotistical, this is a powerful way of disclosing more of themselves to the followers. Even if a supporter does not totally agree with or fully value a leader's mission statement, understanding between the two still increases.

An individual without a sense of purpose is like a rudderless ship—buffeted about by every strong wind that happens along.

People without purpose do not make good leaders. It is difficult, if not impossible, to lead if the individual has no inner sense of direction or understanding of purpose. And in our tumultuous, rapidly changing times, simply adopting someone else's purpose because doing so is politically correct or expedient is not enough. There must be a strong inner sense of knowing and a connection to this identified purpose, or it does not serve during stressful times.

Aligning Missions

This clarity of personal purpose enables leaders to determine whether or not there is a match with their organization. If the organization's purpose or mission is diametrically opposed to a leader's purpose, he or she may feel that carrying out his or her mission is not possible. If encouraging and nurturing followers to function independently and interdependently is part of a leader's mission statement but the leader is in a bureaucratic, heavily hierarchical organization within which there is no intention of empowering employees, this leader would have difficulty feeling successful. Or if a leader sees his or her primary purpose as developing others but recent expansions in scope of responsibility have made it difficult, if not impossible, to serve as a coach for others in the workplace, this role may no longer meet the leader's primary purpose.

Exemplary health care leaders today demonstrate an abiding sense of personal and organizational purpose. Many see themselves as stewards for health care in their communities. Chawla and Renesch (1995) describe this as a willingness for leaders and managers within health care organizations to be accountable for the well-being of the larger community by operating in service to colleagues, patients, families, and other stakeholders. This enduring sense of operating for the benefit of others and for something bigger than any individual helps create committed partnerships with followers. Robert Greenleaf describes it this way in the collection of his private writings, *On Becoming a Servant-Leader* (Frick and Spears, 1996, p. 2):

The servant-leader is servant first. . . . It begins with the
natural feeling that one wants to serve, to serve first.
Then conscious choice brings one to aspire to lead. . . .
The difference manifests itself in the care taken by the
servant—first to make sure that other people's highest-
priority needs are being served. The best test, and the
most difficult to administer, is: Do those served grow as
persons? Do they, while being served, become healthier,
wiser, freer, more autonomous, more likely themselves to
become servants? And, what is the effect on the least
privileged in society; will they benefit or, at least, not be
further deprived?

Vision

The third step for building normative commitment among followers
is through development of a shared vision. In recent years *vision* has
become a byword in management and leadership circles. Everywhere, managers and leaders are exhorted to have a vision. We see
example after example of governments, organizations, and people
for whom vision made a difference. And all are impressive. Joel
Barker in *The Power of Vision* (1990) raises the question: Does vision
come first; or does the success of an individual, organization, or government lead to a vision? In each instance he examined, the vision
came first, leading him to conclude that "vision has the power to
change our lives."

All leaders understand vision because of its presence in their
lives. Vision may not be a concept that is easy to explain, but leaders relate to this idea because they have experienced it. They see
the future differently than other people do: leaders see what is possible and dream, while others merely predict. Vision is really hope
for the future and is based in optimism. It is the ability to rise out
of the current daily turmoil and see something different for the days
and years ahead.

The leader's vision is not necessarily accurate, but it is almost always desirable and positive. Leaders who inspire others with a future vision follow these three crucial steps:

1. Define and describe the vision
2. Engage in dialogue about the vision
3. Create a structure for the vision

The first involves describing the vision; the second is talking about it with others who must help create the new future; and the final step is putting a structure in place to ensure realization of the vision.

Step One: Define and Describe the Vision

A future vision is a picture the leader has of the horizon. The power of vision is in its expectancy; it's a picture of a preferred future, rather than a forecast of a predicted future. Peter Drucker has been credited with saying "the best way to predict the future is to invent it" (Cooper, 1999). Rather than what might be anticipated, it is a desirable future to be sought. It is an illuminated look into tomorrow based on what the leader believes is possible. Vision takes imagination and optimism. "It is the ability to see beyond our present reality, to create, to invent what does not yet exist, to become what we are not yet. It gives us capacity to live out of our imagination instead of our memory" (Covey, Merrill, and Merrill, 1994, pp. 103–104).

Some leaders seek or rise to a leadership position because they have a vision of what the future could be, a vision that drives and inspires them to lead. Armed with the vision, the leader's work of putting structures in place to achieve the desired future becomes simple. Sometimes the position comes first, whether it is a formal leadership position in an organization, appointment to chair a com-

mittee or task force, or election to an office. The individual dis-
covers that he or she has the responsibility and obligation to take
the lead in a situation. Perhaps there is a clear mission but only a
general vision of the outcomes.

The first step is to develop the vision, but this may be more difficult than it sounds. Like the process of creativity, using a deliberate intuitive process is valuable. The intuitive process starts with
preparation by coming to understand as much as possible through
reading anything and everything related to the situation, talking
with people, and drawing on past experiences. The second step is
to let all information and ideas incubate until a spark occurs, leading to illumination, the third step. As the vision becomes clear, it
is important to create as much detail as possible. Concrete, specific
descriptions of a preferred future help others see the vision as well.
John F. Kennedy, when speaking of the U.S. space program in his
1961 state of the union address, did not say: "We will be the world
leaders in space exploration." Instead, he said that before the end
of the decade, the United States would have a man on the moon
and return him safely to Earth. His vision was explicit and definite.

To be inspiring, the preferred future must be a stretch, a far reach
from the present. Martin Luther King Jr. said, "I have a dream that
one day this nation will rise up and live out the true meaning of this
creed—we hold these truths to be self-evident: that all men are created equal" (Anderson, 1990, p. 11). At the time, in segregated
America, this was a tremendous stretch from the reality. Peter Senge
(1990) says that once a vision is identified, the greater the distance
it is from the current reality, the more creative tension exists. Creative tension is the pull between the vision and the present. This
tension acts like a giant rubber band, pulling toward a new future.
During the growth toward a new future, if the new future seems
impossible, it is just too distant; Senge says it is better to extend
time frames than to compromise the vision. Settling for less is the
first step toward mediocrity.

Step Two: Engage in Dialogue about the Vision

A leader alone cannot achieve the vision. New realities are created when everyone whom the vision affects works together. A successful organization or association encourages multiple leaders and in the same way recognizes the need for multiple visions. These visions are more influential if they are consistent, forming a cascade of visions in the organization, as illustrated in Figure 3.2. Everyone has his or her own vision of the future, and a shared vision is created when people engage in dialogue about the vision. They discuss, explore, and modify their visions based on what they learn from each other. A shared vision occurs when two or more people have a similar picture for the future and are each committed to having the vision.

Senge (1990, p. 206) writes, "Today, 'vision' is a familiar concept in corporate leadership. But when you look carefully you find that most 'visions' are one person's (or group's) vision imposed on an organization. Such visions, at best, command compliance—not commitment. A shared vision is a vision that many people are truly committed to, because it reflects their own personal vision." When the shared vision reflects these personal visions, there is a

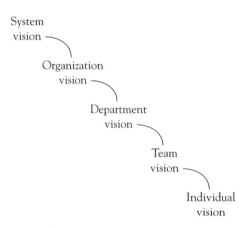

Figure 3.2. A Cascade of Visions

deep sense of caring about reaching the future. Senge describes this shared vision: "A shared vision is not an idea. It is not even an important idea such as freedom. It is, rather, a force in people's hearts, a force of impressive power. It may be inspired by an idea, but once it goes further—if it is compelling enough to acquire the support of more than one person—then it is no longer an abstraction. It is palpable. People begin to see it as if it exists. Few, if any, forces in human affairs are as powerful as shared vision."

Shared visions do not happen unless there is plenty of dialogue about the future. There needs to be open give-and-take, honest questioning, and stimulating conversation about the vision. Abraham Lincoln is a wonderful example of a leader who understood and applied this concept. "Throughout the war Lincoln continued to visit his generals and troops. . . . He always had a kind word for them, frequently telling them his vision of America and how important they were in achieving victory in the cause for which they were fighting" (Phillips, 1992, p. 19).

Step Three: Create a Structure for the Vision

Although Martin Luther King Jr. said "I have a dream" and not "I have a plan," it is not enough to have a dream without a structure in place to ensure the new reality is achieved. To quote the Noah principle: "No more prizes for predicting rain; prizes only for building arks!" The ark in this case is the structure that enables attainment of the desired vision. Some people are great dreamers but are unskilled when it comes to implementing those dreams. Leaders need both skills. "Leaders not only have a vision, they work unusually hard to execute it well. Leaders are implementers, not just strategists; doers, not just dreamers" (Berry, 1992, pp. 2–3). Structure includes the steps to be taken to create the future. A person can dream of winning the lottery, but if he or she never purchases a ticket, the dream never comes true.

Bennis and Nanus (1985) describe vision as the management of attention, and with this simple statement, he captures the power of vision. With a clearly articulated vision and followers who believe in it, the vision itself focuses the attention of the vision community. It keeps people focused on the future, hopeful and expectant about its possibilities. "A leader envisions the destination their followers want, they have the superior skill to guide the journey, and they have the belief to drive the group forward in the face of adversity" (Fagiano, 1994, p. 4).

Shared values, a common purpose or mission, and a shared vision together produce the ability to influence others. An individual leader's personal and deeply held values influence the direction or mission chosen. And a strong sense of mission creates the possibility of commanding visions powerful enough to forge a new future.

Case Example 1: Creating an Integrated Health Care System—The Power of a Collective Vision

Altru Health Systems in Grand Forks, North Dakota, is a fine example of the power of collective vision. In the late 1980s, seven independent entities shared Medical Park, a beautiful campus in central Grand Forks. These entities included an acute-care hospital, a thriving family practice business, a state-owned and -operated rehabilitation hospital, a large primary-care multispeciality medical practice, an orthopedic medical practice, a long-term care facility, and a chemical dependency recovery center. Even in the earliest days, key community leaders foresaw the need to locate all community health services on a jointly shared campus.

The original vision for integration was developed through hospital board retreats held in 1989. The retreats included administrative and medical staff leadership as well as community board members. Armed with this vision, discussions with staff and key stakeholders began. Dialogue revolved around the current reality, future vision, and open discussion about barriers to achieving this vision. Regional stakeholders' initial reactions to the possibility of integrating the hospital and clinic (medical practice) were skeptical. These organizations did not want to be acquired; their autonomy was important to them. Although they agreed they needed to plan together and cooperate, they did not see full integration as a desirable option. Many of the regional organizations expressed the fear that United Hospital and the Grand Forks Clinic would buy up and close the smaller organizations in an attempt to reduce competition. Both United Hospital and the Grand Forks Clinic assured them that they would not go into their community without an invitation.

From these discussions, the involved leaders developed a strong belief that integrating the facilities in Medical Park would be a necessary first step. If integration could not be successful there, it could not be attained in the region. This helped formulate strategies to reach the vision. Based on these dialogues, the parties established concrete strategies for achieving the vision in early 1990, projecting that they would attain the vision in the year 2000. United Hospital's board of directors held their CEO, Rosemary Jacobson, accountable by requiring from her a thrice-annual review of progress against these strategies.

A persistent win-win approach helped overcome resistance and created increasing buy-in to the vision of a fully integrated health care system for the community. Over the years the groups overcame barriers, and strategies were successful. They reached agreement regarding the need to have common governance, a common bottom line, and integrated operations. By 1995 the family medicine and orthopedic practices had been integrated with the Grand Forks Clinic, and the chemical dependency recovery center and rehabilitation hospital were integrated into United Hospital. Final steps were being taken to integrate Grand Forks Clinic with United Health Services. Other entities were asked to join, and Pathology Associates joined in 1996.

The last step to integrating the clinic and hospital was the most difficult. Board and executive leaderships of both organizations were fully committed to the vision, but many physicians at the clinic were skeptical or opposed to the initiative. Both organizations were financially successful, so they had no strong fiscal incentives to pursue integration. Both were concerned about the profound effects of combining their cultures. The boards of directors in each organization were fully committed to their internal staff and were committed to few or no layoffs. There was a clear expectation, however, that cross training, modification of roles, and new assignments would occur as operations became integrated. The integration displaced few individuals. Work areas and roles were altered, and working relationships were disrupted. The difference in cultures was measured and found not to be as different as anticipated. The two "new" organizations entered the final eighteen months of negotiation in a state of some stress. Without true commitment to this shared vision, the journey would have been impossible.

These months were difficult and at times discouraging. Rosemary Jacobson, then president and CEO of United Health Services (which included United Hospital), believed that the unwavering support, commitment, and stubborn persistence on the part of executive and board leadership at both facilities were the catalysts for surviving those final months. The chairman of the hospital board attended 99 percent of the integration meetings, and his commitment and openness were instrumental in allaying fears of community control of the clinic and physician practices. Even in the face of direct opposition, the leadership of both organizations stayed true to the collective vision they shared. Potential personal losses were also an issue. Both CEOs realized they had to share the commitment to this vision to ensure good access to health care in their region, or their health care system would be damaged. Initially, the two CEOs brought experience from both the clinic and hospital side of the business.

Noteworthy throughout this process was the absence of external consultants. The organizations engaged outside attorneys to ensure that they considered all legal ramifications, but otherwise organizational leadership fully managed the process. Ms. Jacobson noted: "It took more courage and guts than brains!" Retaining control of, responsibility for, and active involvement in the process created a tremendous sense of ownership on the part of leadership in these organizations.

The closing stages were characterized by starts and stops, intense communication, discouragement, stalemates, and periods when both parties withdrew from the negotiations. Finally, a growing momentum resulted in attainment of the vision a full three years ahead of schedule. United Health Services and Grand Forks Clinic became officially integrated on July 1, 1997. This accomplishment is even more significant when one remembers that this community was devastated by a cripplingly destructive spring flood that year, following one of the most difficult winters in the city's history. Even as the community was struggling to cope with its overwhelming losses and restore adequate living conditions, its health care leaders were looking to the future. The power of a shared vision had transformed health care in this region.

Ms. Jacobson credited the successful attainment of this vision to repeated and continual dialogue and communication about the vision, a commitment to listening and responding to reactions, perseverance in spite of naysayers, and a level of commitment among key leaders to a mission that extended well beyond their own interests. The formulation of a shared vision provided the impetus and direction to develop strategies that helped achieve the vision. Ms. Jacobson said of the vision: "It enabled us to make progress, where otherwise we wouldn't have." The leaders of this change were trustworthy individuals serving as stewards for their community. Each leader was absolutely committed to a shared vision of full access to the highest quality of health care services for the community and region they serve. Multiple champions working in concert were essential to the effort's success.

Today the system is fully operational with structural components for the system integrated. A physician president and administrator CEO work in partnership to lead the entity. At the operational level, physician and administrative leaders work in partnership to provide day-to-day oversight. Although the issue of physician alignment remains a challenge, increasing numbers of physicians are now involved in organizational strategic visioning and planning. And patient-care outcomes and employee satisfaction levels are high. In the midst of significant national nursing shortages, the organization enjoys only a 2 percent vacancy rate and uses no travelers (workers from outside the community with short-term assignments) and limited temporary employees. The result of this far-reaching vision affects the quality of health care in the entire region.

Case Example 2: Improving the Delivery of Care– A Department Leader's Vision

The scope of this case example is more limited than the development of an integrated health care system but no less significant in terms of its impact on the people being served. It involved Joan, a director of maternal-child nursing in a five hundred–bed community hospital in a western state. (She prefers to remain anonymous.) Her areas of responsibility included six patient-care departments: labor and delivery, postpartum, newborn nursery, neonatal intensive care, and two pediatric units. When Joan was recruited to this organization, these departments were managed in a traditional fashion and were gradually declining in market share because their maternity services were basically unresponsive to customers' requests.

Joan had been in her position for three years and was well respected throughout the organization for her innovative leadership style. During those three years, she had established good relationships with employees in the various departments and had gradually hired new managers who more closely shared her values of employee empowerment and participatory leadership as well as family-centered maternity care. In spite of a traditional medical staff and administration who preferred to maintain the status quo, Joan held a vision of a women's service in which care was organized around the family unit instead of segregated into four different departments.

As Joan and her new managers began implementing innovative programs and services, the hospital's market share for obstetrics began slowly regaining ground. After three years the service was bursting at the seams, requiring more postpartum beds and bassinet space. The closest patient-care area available was a rehabilitation department in the next wing of the hospital. An expansion was planned for an additional ten postpartum beds and a small nursery for newborns to be added to the maternity unit. However, this new patient-care unit was so small that staffing would be a significant problem unless employees were cross trained to care for either mother or baby. Suddenly, Joan's long-held vision for a mother-and-baby unit was possible. Commitment to this vision began with frequent discussions with all stakeholders. Employees, managers, and physicians were all involved in planning discussions. Major educational sessions were offered to introduce the concept to key stakeholders.

In several instances, commitment was difficult to gain because people involved held values that differed from Joan's belief in maintaining the integrity of the family unit. Additionally, this change represented a major impact on postpartum and newborn nursery employees, many of whom believed they could not handle the change. A planning committee of employees and physicians worked out details for the expansion unit. Employees volunteered and were then selected and trained. The implementation process proceeded smoothly, and within months the department had a waiting list of expectant parents. Demand for this service was so intense that the hospital converted the original postpartum unit to mother-and-baby care two years later.

This example may not seem remarkable except that it took place in the early 1980s, long before mother-and-baby care was the norm for women and newborn services. In fact, this was the first such conversion in a region of several states and is today continuing to provide true family-centered care for those it serves. It started with one individual's vision but became possible only when those within the vision community shared the vision. Together they created a powerful new reality that improved health care in the area.

Case Example 3: Vision Failed

Successfully attaining a vision creates tremendous feelings of pride and accomplishment for the individuals involved. There is optimism for the future, and people see the direction they are headed. In this final example, however, the outcomes were not positive. Individuals made errors in judgment, and the results actually damaged the organization's viability.

This is the story of a large community hospital in the mid-1990s. The CEO had been reading about vision and believed a clear vision was needed within his organization. He assigned two interested and capable individuals within the organization as consultants to develop a vision statement. They interviewed the CEO and one or two other key executives to gather ideas and concepts, then worked hard to develop a positive stretch vision from these ideas. The first draft of the vision statement was beautifully worded and certainly far-reaching, and it seemed to be the direction the organization was already heading. The two internal consultants met with the executive leadership group to share this vision and engage in dialogue about it. This step was only moderately successful because the discussion was somewhat stilted and limited. However, the group identified strategies for sharing the vision with employees, with the next step to include holding focus-group discussions.

Based on input from these focus groups, the consultants made minor changes in the vision. But most important was the concern that managers and employees alike raised, relating skepticism and doubt about executive commitment to this vision. This response and concern fell on deaf ears. The CEO disregarded advice from the two consultants. The internal consultants prepared the final draft and presented it at a department managers' meeting, with beautiful over-heads and fine rhetoric. Empowered employees and conversion to a team-based organization formed the foundation of the vision. The consultants concretely presented the terms with many fine examples. However, there was limited buy-in from anyone in the organization.

Four years later the organization had undergone repeated crises, internal conflicts, a successful union organizing attempt, and the stressful effects of a rapidly changing external environment. Where other organizations' vision of a new future had guided them through turbulent times, this organization emerged weaker and more disor-ganized than it was before the development of the vision. What was the problem? At least three factors prevented the attainment of the vision. The first was the CEO's mistakenly held but strong belief that the organization should have only one vision. Over the years he and members of his executive group had discouraged the development of additional, congruent visions by individuals and teams, preferring that the only vision in use be the organization's vision statement. The organization actively discouraged departments and work groups from developing their own vision to fit within the organization's vision. The end result was a preponderance of individuals and teams who saw the organization's vision statement as administrative rhetoric that did not directly apply to them or their team.

A second factor was the executives' unwillingness to consistently model their behavior on the very behavior they expected from employees. Highly visible examples of the old command-and-control approach to management continued to occur in spite of the language in the vision statement about valuing employee empowerment. And the executives never got around to developing themselves as a team, although the vision clearly expected participation in teams from all employees. The final nail in the coffin was the internal managers' lack of commitment to the vision. Most of the communication about the vision came from the internal consultants rather than the CEO. Even though the vision sounded great, the managers were cynical about the possibility of ever attaining it. Over time those employees who

were initially committed to the vision felt betrayed, which caused cynicism that became quite virulent about what they felt was a bogus
vision statement.

Common Pitfalls

Leadership interventions for strengthening employee organizational
commitment seem relatively straightforward. However, as with any
issue dealing with human behavior and interactions, there are often
hidden pitfalls and challenges to be considered. Several of the most
common issues are addressed here.

Mistaking Compliance for Commitment

Effective leaders grasp the difference between commitment and
compliance and do not mistake one for the other. Leadership is
more than influencing others to follow a specific direction; it is creating a desire within the followers to do so. This chapter briefly
discussed compliance earlier. Because most leaders also have the
legitimate authority of a position, they may be tempted to rely on
giving others direction about the needed actions and behaviors.

At first glance, it may seem easier to seek compliance rather
than invest in the preparation time to build commitment. Simply
telling people what to do and expecting conformance takes less
time. The time it takes to gain commitment is illustrated in Figure
3.3. The arrow indicates a project, decision, or action that must be
implemented. The preparation time for gaining compliance is relatively short, whereas gaining commitment requires a long, intense
preparatory period of lengthy conversations, exploration of shared
values, dialogue about purpose, open sharing of information, and
collaborative development of the vision and plan. All of these steps
lead to the internal shift within the person that indicates a deep
level of commitment to the outcome (illustrated by the longer line
before implementation).

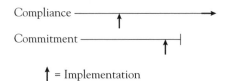

↑ = Implementation

Figure 3.3. Comparing Compliance and Commitment in Terms of Time Investment

The paradox, of course, is that if leaders provide thorough preparation and treat employees as partners on the journey, the attainment of the desired outcome is actually much faster. In many instances in which organizations seek mere compliance, leaders find they have created an open-ended process with no closure because there are always some who do not comply (as seen with the open-ended compliance line). They simply have not bought in to the concept and do not support it. Unfortunately, it does not take many of these people within your group to sabotage and undermine the vision. And in too many cases, the resistant behavior may be covert and not readily apparent. In either case, full compliance and closure is never attained. A strong leader understands the difference between compliance and commitment and consciously decides when commitment is needed and when compliance is enough.

Failing to Offer Choice in the Work Environment

When leaders understand commitment, the importance of choice in making a commitment is clear. Brickman, Wortman, and Sorrentino's construct of commitment (1987) indicates that commitment includes a positive element, a negative element, and a bond between the two. This implies that there are alternatives to be considered and evaluated. If there is no choice, there is really no commitment because there are not two elements between which a bond is formed. Thus, choice is essential to the concept of commitment. The opportunity of choice is an important construct in American culture: "For Americans . . . making a choice provides an opportunity to display one's preferences and, consequently, to express one's internal attributes, to assert one's autonomy, and to fulfill the goal of being unique" (Iyengar and Lepper, 1999, p. 350).

"Choice is crucial to commitment" (Waterman, 1987, p. 299). Employees choose whether or not to commit and follow the path indicated. Commitment cannot be forced, and this means that a leader must face the possibility that people may choose *not* to follow. Waterman writes: "If the most competent and trusted people won't commit, the leader should take another look at the cause itself. It may be ill-conceived or stated in a misleading way" (p. 299). And forcing a choice prematurely is risky. Leaders must be comfortable with employees making their own choices in their own time about the commitments they make because once people have made a choice, research has demonstrated, they are less open to new information (Brickman, Wortman, and Sorrentino, 1987). People need more information in order to change a decision than to make one. Demanding compliance on a course of action that requires employees' full engagement and support is hazardous because it may preclude the possibility of ever achieving true commitment.

Probably the most important ramification in providing choice has to do with understanding why emphasizing continuance commitment is so damaging. If the salary and benefits levels are high, the employee perceives fewer alternatives; that is, leaving the organization costs too much. An employee who feels trapped, even by positive circumstances, is less likely to be positively engaged. So although competitive compensation packages are desirable, other rewards such as job variety, promotion opportunities, increased autonomy, and coworker support are probably more effective (Iverson and Buttigieg, 1999).

Insufficient Communication

Recognizing that making a commitment is a rational decision-making process underscores the critical importance of communication. Information is crucial in any decision-making process, for it forms the basis on which one makes the decision. This relates back to the recommendation that there be an open flow of information about the leader's and employee's individual values and mission as well as the organization's values and mission. Involving employees in developing a shared vision of what this venture will look like in the future helps create enthusiasm and commitment. Honest and sincere dialogue between a leader and followers helps further shape and enhance the direction. As Senge (1990) pointed out, only when the vision is shared is true commitment to and engagement with it possible.

How do we get from thought to action? The choices may seem overwhelming. Rational decision making requires accurate information. What are the alternatives? What are the consequences of choosing different alternatives? "The essential conflict between rational thought and functional behavior can be put very simply. Rational thought requires consideration of all available alternatives. Effective action requires the pursuit of one alternative, not necessarily the best one, and the ignoring or suppressing of the others" (Brickman, Wortman, and Sorrentino, 1987, p. 51). Decisions must be made and action taken even if compelling arguments exist on both sides of the issue. Being rational means that an individual chooses the best alternative. Thus, a key issue in rationality is whether the individual is aware of the alternatives and his or her reasons for choosing one above the other.

The influence of a commitment needs to be respected. "To whatever extent people are rational, they are less so following commitment" (Brickman, Wortman, and Sorrentino, 1987, p. 35). When circumstances result in the dissolution of commitments, especially those we have asked people to make, we cannot expect a rapid resolution to the emotions involved. A recent example illustrates this. In a small Georgia community, two hospitals with a long history of fierce competition were set on a course to merge. The CEOs in each facility worked diligently to gain the commitment of employees, physicians, and community. Their strongest argument was that this course of action was the only hope for survival of both facilities.

People were convinced and became quite committed to the merger. Imagine the difficulties when the merger fell through!

Missing the Possibility of Escalating Commitment

Another key aspect that effective leaders understand is the concept of escalating commitment. This social psychology concept is related to our need for self-justification. "Escalation is self-perpetuating. Once a small commitment is made, it sets the stage for ever-increasing commitments. The behavior needs to be justified, so attitudes are changed; this change in attitudes influences future decisions and behaviors" (Aronson, 1995, p. 192). This is why many savvy telemarketers begin by asking a question to which the person answering the telephone can respond only positively. It sets you up for a positive second response. Similarly, if a leader can get even a small commitment first, it sets the stage for more significant commitments later.

Conclusion

Compliance from followers is not enough during these difficult and demanding times. Exemplary leaders build among followers commitments to a certain course of action. Such leaders also understand the different forms of organizational commitment and know how to capitalize on these to create a positive work environment. Effective leaders focus their efforts predominantly on building affective and normative organizational commitment. Shared values, a mission common and relevant to all, and a shared vision are three specific ways in which a leader can build normative commitment among followers. Affective organizational commitment occurs when healthy relationships and a strong sense of connection exist between people in the workplace. When these two forms of commitment are present, employees do not just comply with directions set by those leaders but want to follow the path. Together these things inspire passion and provide the energy and courage to create a new reality.

Sometimes we have to believe in something before we can visualize it. And it won't materialize until it is believed.

Conversation Points

1. Think of something to which you are committed. How did your commitment begin? What has kept it strong over time? What are the elements of your commitment? Which is the positive element, and which is the negative?

2. Which form of organizational commitment (continuance, affective, normative) do you think is the strongest in your organization?

3. What are your most important work-related values? Ask yourself: "What do I stand for? How do I treat my coworkers or colleagues? What do I mean by ethical behavior? How do I want to be known by others?"

4. Once you have a list of your important values, identify the specific day-to-day behaviors you engage in that demonstrate that you live by these values. Are there gaps between what you say you value and how you live your life? What values do you say you hold but find you don't express frequently enough? What values do you neglect during periods of high stress?

5. Think of an example when you had to decide which values were more important. What was the situation, and how did you resolve it? In retrospect, did you make the right decision? Would you change that decision today?

6. What can you do to ensure that you are living by your values each day?

7. What is your personal and your leadership mission? Why are you here? What do you do, and for whom do you do it? Take some time to reflect and write a personal and a leadership mission statement.

8. What is your future vision? Where do you see yourself in five years? What will you be doing? How will you get there?

9. Consider your organization's values, mission, and vision statement. Are your values, mission, and vision congruent with those of your department, service, or organization?

10. Find someone whose vision has made a difference in their life. Ask them to share their story.

4

Communicating with Clarity

The greatest problem of communication is the illusion
that it has been accomplished.

George Bernard Shaw

The ability to communicate clearly is essential to excelling as a leader. Efforts to establish a leadership relationship, build commitment, manage processes, and develop others are futile without superior communication skills. Although some people believe that simply being articulate is enough, there is far more to proficient communication. Good leaders cultivate openness in their communication; they believe followers desire and deserve information pertaining to their work. Exceptional leaders have a high degree of emotional intelligence competencies, one of the most important being the ability to communicate not just information but emotion. They clearly recognize that through their communication they establish connections with others (Kowalski and Yoder-Wise, 2003).

This chapter tackles the issue of sharing information openly and explores several communication techniques for leadership effectiveness. It reviews common barriers to effective communication and offers ideas for overcoming them. It also presents special issues in leadership communication. Many people overestimate the ease of meeting this competency because it appears to be simple, and almost everyone has attended some kind of communication course or seminar. Managers and leaders today spend more of their time communicating than ever before, yet the most common complaints from followers concern communication: "We don't get enough information"; "Nobody is telling us anything"; and "Communication here is rotten."

Exacerbating the problem are those individuals who overestimate their effectiveness at communicating. "A few individuals may exhibit exceptional interpersonal skills, a great many others may demonstrate weak, negative, or virtually nonexistent interpersonal skills. Such considerable difficulty as we know exists . . . because most individuals do not believe there is anything wrong with the way they communicate face-to-face. . . . Most persons inherently believe they are better communicators than they actually are" (McConnell, 2004, p. 177). These people believe that if they open their mouths and words flow out or they have sent a memo or made an announcement, communication has occurred. This leads to a false sense of security and sometimes an attitude of arrogance: "I've communicated; if they didn't get it, that's their problem." Perhaps nothing destroys the leader's effectiveness as quickly as a lack of information and miscommunication. Distrust rapidly grows, and the leader's credibility shrinks.

Communication is a necessary component of emotional competency. The effectiveness of our relationship skills hinges on our ability not only to attune ourselves to or influence another person's emotions but also to take this knowledge into account when we communicate. Emotionally intelligent leaders who exhibit a communication competency "are effective in the give-and-take of emotional information, deal with difficult issues straightforwardly, listen well and welcome sharing information fully, foster open communication and stay receptive to bad news as well as good" (Cherniss and Goleman, 2001, p. 37). A healthy and open dialogue depends on the leader staying attuned to others' emotional states and controlling their own impulses to respond in ways that might impair or restrict open communication.

Defining Communication

Communication is the act of interchanging or imparting thoughts, opinions, ideas, emotions, or information by speech, writing, or other signs. It has been described as the flow of information from a sender to a receiver by way of a channel (Figure 4.1.). The channel might be verbal, the written or spoken word, or nonverbal, such as body language or the environment. When the receiver gets the message and experiences the same meaning that the sender understands, communication is complete. The sender may either perceive a change in the receiver's behavior or hear that the receiver has received the message, and this feedback closes the communication loop.

Common Problems

As simple as it may seem, the communication loop model contains multiple problematic areas. A skilled communicator understands these potential problems and takes steps to avert them when possible.

Noise

Noise anywhere in the system can reduce the likelihood of transferring a message accurately. Noise is more than loud or distracting sounds that impair the ability to hear. It can be anything that reduces the ability to receive the message accurately, including the

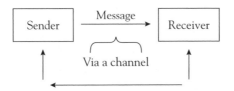

Figure 4.1. The Communication Loop Model

state of the receiver's body or mind (the presence of tension, anxiety, or any intense emotion), elements that cloud the message (jargon, words with multiple meanings, assumptions, and biases), and
attitudes of the receiver toward the message (perhaps the message
is something the receiver does not want to hear or has prejudged).

Choice of Channel

Another potential problem area is the choice of channel. Announc-
ing major organization changes by memo rather than face-to-face
communication may send the wrong message. Changing channels
unexpectedly can affect the message's clarity. If the usual channel
between the sender and the receiver is the face-to-face spoken word,
switching to a formal written memo can add emphasis. If the message is negative, the change in channel may so accentuate its tone
that it raises exaggerated emotions in the receiver, making a correct
interpretation of that message difficult.

John, the manager of environmental services, and Mary, the
manager of a patient-care department, found themselves in this
kind of situation. They communicated frequently, mostly talking
face-to-face, about issues and problems related to the environmental services function in the patient-care area. In the previous year,
there had been repeated problems because of the increased responsibilities assigned to the environmental service workers. Mary, frustrated after a particularly bad day, sent John a memo outlining
unresolved problems. Because she was irritated, she also sent a copy
to John's supervisor.

John felt blasted by the memo as well as betrayed because Mary
also sent it to his supervisor. The memo contained nothing that
they hadn't talked about before, but the channel selection accen-
tuated the message dramatically and almost destroyed John's willingness to cooperate further with Mary. Even though most leaders
are aware of these basic principles, it is still easy to get caught up in
a situation and make a poor judgment. Leaders need patience to
persevere in the face of these challenges.

Responsibility

Another potential problem is the issue of responsibility. Although the receiver has some responsibility to respond to the message received, the sender retains full responsibility for the message until the feedback loop is closed. If the sender gets feedback that the message was not received clearly, it is the sender's responsibility to resend the message, perhaps modifying it in a way that increases the likelihood of understanding. If no feedback is forthcoming, the sender seeks a response that is appropriate to the situation, for example: What did you understand me to say? Have you acted on the information in the memo? What action have you taken? Communication is a covenant between sender and receiver, and too often the sender believes that once the message has gone out, the sender's responsibility ends.

Feedback

On concrete, tangible issues, feedback may result from observing the receiver's reaction or behavior after receiving the message. Perhaps the worst mistake the sender can make, however, is to assume that because the message was sent, the responsibility has shifted to the receiver. As a result, the sender does not follow up, makes the assumption that all is well, and then blames the receiver when events do not go as the sender intended.

We see this regularly: a written memo or e-mail message goes out, but only half the people who were supposed to receive it ever do. For example, the education department notifies potential participants of an upcoming program for which they need to register, but the memo doesn't make it to all intended recipients. Those who do not receive the message may appear resistant or negative because they do not take the required action or as complaining if they point out that they were left out of the loop. E-mail has contributed to this problem because it leaves no paper trail unless the communicator intentionally creates one. We quickly tap out messages and instantly distribute them with a single keystroke to multiple recipients. But the old adage "Out of sight, out of mind" holds true. It is difficult to remember to follow up on something if we have no reminders!

If the relationship with receivers is not built on trust, the feedback the sender gets may not be entirely honest. The receiver may be embarrassed to admit that the memo, proposal, or vision statement was so filled with buzzwords, jargon, ten-letter words, highly technical language, or just plain gobbledygook that the receiver really did not understand what it said. The receiver may also find it difficult to admit that he or she did not get the message the first time because of distractions in the environment. Or perhaps the sender responded in an angry and defensive fashion when the receiver gave negative feedback on a previous occasion, and the receiver is not willing to endure such a response again. Trust in the sender is essential for accurate feedback to occur.

When feedback is negative, a common assumption is that the receiver has an attitude problem. The conclusion may be that the person receiving the message purposely did not take the intended action and is being obstructive, resistive, or just plain stupid. Instead, to avoid this pitfall, the first question the sender might ask is whether there were technical or semantic problems with the communication. The sender must consider these first before assuming that the receiver has an attitude problem.

Case Example 1: Miscommunication

A parenting example makes the distinctions between different communication problems clearer. A family expects overnight company during the weekend, and on Wednesday the parents of sixteen-year-old Sarah ask her to clean her room so that the visitors can sleep in it. Friday arrives, and Sarah has not cleaned her room. A typical parental reaction is to assume that Sarah just didn't get around to it, didn't follow through, or was perhaps being rebellious in reaction to giving up her room or being told what to do (an attitude problem).

If Mom looks back, however, to see how she carried out her responsibility as sender, she might find other reasons for the miscommunication. For instance, she may remember that when she told Sarah to clean her room, Sarah was on her way out the door. Also, Sarah had stayed up late studying for a test she was very worried about, and she had overslept and was late leaving for school (internal anxiety—noise in the system). And as any parent knows, "Clean your room" may mean one thing to a sixteen-year-old and something entirely different to a parent (semantic differences). To Sarah, it meant getting everything out of sight: stuffed under the bed or in the drawers or the closet. To her mom, it meant emptying a drawer and making closet space available, as well as assuring that odors and clutter emanating from under the bed wouldn't disturb the guests.

Case Example 2: Mixed Messages

Similar examples exist in the work world. A three hundred-bed hospital in the St. Louis area was in severe financial straits. Part of a larger system, the hospital was given six months to reverse these financial problems or the facility would be sold. The director of education purchased modular education that the managers and supervisors (as internal facilitators) were to deliver to employees in the belief that this education would assist in an extensive downsizing and restructuring effort that was under way. An outside trainer arrived to present the modules for the internal facilitators beginning on a Monday afternoon.

On Monday morning the internal facilitators were gathered together and received a message from the CEO regarding the corporate decision about a likely closure or sale, a planned layoff, and the reduction of management and supervisory positions by half. In the afternoon these same people were expected to attend a learning and development session! Even though these people rallied and concentrated on how they could use the educational modules, the effectiveness of any communication that afternoon was greatly reduced by the presence of strong emotions (a technical problem) following the morning session. If administrators later labeled these managers and supervisors as resistant or nonsupportive because they had not used the modules, this example would closely parallel the parenting example in the previous case example.

Case Example 3: Inappropriate Settings

A management development specialist told the story of feedback she received from her leader regarding an important project that the leader had asked her to undertake. Their offices were located in different cities in the same state, making face-to-face feedback difficult because of inaccessibility. It happened that both the specialist and the leader were attending a seminar together. The specialist decided to use this opportunity to obtain feedback on the project, but the only place and time available was in the women's rest room during a break. As one might imagine, the feedback left a lot to be desired.

How many important conversations take place in the hallway or in the minutes before or after meetings? There never seems to be enough time to communicate thoroughly, and yet the sender and receiver may end up spending hours to clear up miscommunication.

Communication and Leadership

Warren Bennis and Burt Nanus describe communication as the management of meaning (1985). When Max DePree (1989) talks about a leader's role as defining reality, he is referring to the belief that the understanding of the reality is one that the leader and follower share. Shared meaning is the very essence of communication. The leader communicates not only words and concepts throughout the organization but emotional tone as well. One of the most important things the leader communicates is his or her emotions. "Emotions are contagious, particularly when exhibited by those at the top, and extremely successful leaders display a high level of positive energy that spreads throughout the organization" (Cherniss and Goleman, 2001, p. 38). The emotional tone that the leader sets ripples out through the organization and has significant impact.

Although complete and totally accurate communication is probably impossible to attain, a more reasonable goal is to accomplish enough clear communication to enable followers to act on ideas or information in a positive and forward-moving manner. The sender of the message retains responsibility until the receiver closes the feedback loop. Following up on feedback and assessing the message for technical, semantic, or attitude difficulties can prevent major miscues.

Information

Information is one of the most important things we transmit through communication. Information is like a lubricant in the system, and without it the different parts simply do not work well together. In an automobile, if there is not enough oil in the engine, gears grind, friction develops, and overheating can destroy the parts. The same happens in an organization. Margaret Wheatley, in *Leadership and the New Science* (1992), does a beautiful job of exploring the role of information in a system: "If information is not available, people make it up. Rumors proliferate, things get out of hand—all because people lack the real thing. Given the need for constant nourishing information, it is no wonder that 'poor communication' inevitably appears so high on the problems list. Employees know it is the critical vital sign of organizational health" (p. 107).

Part of the problem is that many people regard information as stable, factual, and something that is the same today as it will be tomorrow. Information is instead dynamic and ever changing. Simply sharing it may essentially change the information as it is passed along, much like the childhood game of telephone. "The function of information is revealed in the word itself: in-formation. . . . For a system to remain alive, for the universe to move onward, information must be continually generated. If there is nothing new, or if the information that exists merely confirms what is, then the result will be death" (Wheatley, 1992, p. 104).

Leaders who treat information as something static and fail to appreciate its dynamic quality end up frustrated by the need to continually communicate with others. Followers who see information as stable have great difficulty understanding why the message today is different from the message yesterday. Some followers conclude that the leader was not being honest yesterday or did not have accurate information, because they find it hard to believe that the information could change that quickly. Mistrust grows quickly unless followers understand the true nature of information, that it is always in formation.

The leader's attitude toward sharing information is crucial to being an expert communicator (Wilson, George, and Wellins, 1994). At least five rationales, or internal messages the leader may be playing, affect the amount of information the leader shares with followers:

- Followers already know the information.

- Followers do not want to know.

- Followers do not need to know.

- Followers cannot understand this information.

- Everyone is on information overload.

Followers Already Know the Information

A common misconception that hampers many would-be excellent communicators is the assumption that because they shared the information once, the receiver understood the message. Only a very unusual follower gets the message right the first time. With so much noise in our changing systems and with stress levels as high as they are, it is almost guaranteed that we need to repeat messages multiple times before they are received accurately. In fact, during times of great change in the organization, leaders should expect to repeat messages at least seven to ten times before receivers understand them.

Not only do the messages need to be repeated frequently, but using a variety of different channels will increase the likelihood that they will be received. This means using a combination of channels such as face-to-face dialogues, spoken presentations, written methods, and modeling the behavior we request. The greater the frequency and the wider the variety of methods we use to communicate messages, the more likely they will get through. Another key principle is to encode the message with what it means for the receiver: why it is important and what the impact is on the receiver's life.

Followers Do Not Want to Know

In one organization a benevolent, paternalistic leader's attitude was "They don't really want the truth—they couldn't handle it." Even in a supportive, empowering leader, the thought that the truth would scare the followers can be a deterrent to open communication with them. Some leaders believe that part of their role is to shield followers from bad news. In fact, some followers say: "You take care of that; we don't want to know the gory details." In these cases, followers are giving up their power and sense of control to the leader.

This leader attitude displays a lack of respect for followers. From the leader's perspective, it implies that the followers are not strong enough or able to handle difficult news or unpleasant information. "When we shield people we are acting as their parents and treating them like children" (Block, 1987, p. 91). It is better to err on the side of high expectations of others than to continue to weaken followers' self-esteem by keeping them from the truth.

Followers Do Not Need the Information

In some instances, the leader believes that followers do not need certain information, that it is privileged or confidential. The notion of sharing information openly is the opposite of the military model that "only those that 'need to know' should be informed" (Block, 1987, p. 90). Here's an extreme example from a southwestern community hospital. The executive team in this 320-bed facility spends several weeks each year involved in strategic planning. Team members analyze the organization's strengths, weaknesses, opportunities, and threats and plot out the steps for action over the next two to three years. The team is very clear about its direction and what the hospital needs to do to accomplish the plan's outcomes.

Interestingly, however, the executive team never shares the plan with employees or managers! The team is afraid someone will leak it to the hospital's competitor, a similar-sized facility in the same community. Employees and managers alike have directly and repeatedly asked over the years to see the plan. Many have reached the conclusion that there really is no plan. How this executive team expects to accomplish its strategic plan in isolation from employees and managers is a mystery. This situation has led to significant feelings of mistrust in the organization.

Instead, the goal should be to let followers know of plans, ideas, and changes as soon as possible. Plans cannot be implemented without the support and involvement of followers, who need to be included from the beginning. Robert Haas, quoted in Huey (1994, p. 48), says: "In a command and control organization, people protect knowledge because it's their claim to distinction. But we share as much information as we possibly can throughout the company.

Business literacy is a big issue in developing leadership. You cannot ask people to exercise broader judgment if their world is bounded by very narrow vision."

Followers Cannot Understand the Information

Admittedly, much of the information concerning the health care environment and community issues can be very complex. However, the workforce today is better educated and informed than ever. When Congress was debating U.S. trade agreements some years ago, so were workers on factory-room floors all over this country. Becoming well informed is as simple as turning on a television set. Increased availability of information through mass media has resulted in well-informed citizens—when they choose to seek the information.

Employees or followers are capable of understanding a great deal more than some leaders give them credit for. Increased appreciation for employees' capabilities has been a wonderfully liberating outcome for organizations that have successfully implemented models of shared decision making in their organizations, such as shared governance structures, unit councils, and employee work teams and helped these employees develop to a high level of self-direction and self-management (Manion, Lorimer, and Leander, 1996). Many think that traditional management responsibilities—such as departmental budgeting, interviewing and selecting new employees, planning, and managing supplies and inventory—are beyond the capabilities of the average employee. Yet these same employees leave at the end of their workday and assume these very responsibilities in their homes. They manage financial resources, possibly serve on a church board undertaking a multimillion-dollar building project, help their children select vocational schools or colleges, and resolve conflict within the family. The next morning at work brings sudden dependence on a manager to accomplish very similar tasks.

In a Baltimore hospital, executives discovered the power of sharing increasingly complex information with employees. Over the years the administration had made great strides in creating an empowering environment. Executives shared information openly and freely with employees. The hospital held town hall–style meetings, with executives and employees engaging in direct dialogue about issues of concern. In the early stages of this transformation, the questions employees asked executives at these meetings involved issues such as adequacy of parking space, health care benefits, and expected structural changes. As months passed and the executives shared more information, employee questions changed significantly. Executives began hearing questions such as: What's our managed care penetration? How is progress going on the contract with . . . ? What is the impact of recent legislative changes on our organization and community? The more information the leaders shared, the more sophisticated followers became, and the broader their understanding was of the organization's reality.

Everyone Is Already Overloaded with Information

A common and often justified message playing in a leader's head is that followers are already on overload and too much information is potentially damaging. The leader's concern is that excess information may be overwhelming. There is no question that the overload of information exists and only worsens as each year passes.

No one is immune from the information explosion. The elderly remember days before television when radio was the primary media. Baby boomers remember when only two or three channels were available on television. Now communication is possible virtually anywhere, anytime. Cell telephones, instant messaging, beepers, fax machines, overnight express mail—all contribute to the immediacy of available information. Computers and mass media in addition to voice and electronic mail have contributed to an information glut. It's no wonder everyone feels overloaded. The flow of information is an unrelenting bombardment that continues throughout nearly every waking hour.

A *Wall Street Journal* article (Markels, 1997, p. B1) reports widespread dismay at the number of messages being sent: "The average person sends and receives a total of about 178 messages each day, according to a recent study of 972 workers at large companies." The study also found that this communication barrage causes repeated interruptions of work, leaving people feeling frustrated and overwhelmed. Appreciating this information overload is important, but it should not keep the leader from sharing as much as possible about the project or situation.

The Leader's Primary Responsibilities: Information and Communication

Because of the glut of information in the environment, an effective communicator knows that messages need to be simple and easy to understand. Using a variety of channels helps ensure reception. Analyzing how the information is important to the recipient gives the leader clues about preparing effective transmission.

Communication is a full-time responsibility for all leaders. A leader cannot communicate too much. It is far better to err on the side of excess information even though it may create its own problems at times. "The fuel of life is new information. . . . We need to have information coursing through our systems, disturbing the peace, imbuing everything it touches with new life. We need, therefore, to develop new approaches to information—not management but encouragement, not control but genesis. How do we create more of this wonderful life source?" (Wheatley, 1992, p. 105). Many organizations today have chief information officers to help the system develop an approach to handling the massive amounts of information available. Learning organizations must be able to disseminate information widely in order to learn from all parts of the organization in a timely manner.

A leader must master three methods of communication—spoken, nonverbal, and written—in order to be an effective information disseminator. The more versatile the leader is in these three methods, the more congruent the message and the more likely it will transmit clearly. This section explores principles of each method with ramifications for today's health care leaders. Not all followers are equally skilled as communicators, and the less skilled the follower, the more highly skilled the leader needs to be.

Spoken Communication

Spoken communication is more than selecting the words. For a leader to influence followers, there must be a way to exchange ideas and opinions, to dialogue about issues, and to share concerns. This is usually done through oral communication. Successful communication includes the following aspects:

- Delivering the message clearly

- Creating a message with impact

- Getting the listener's attention

- Establishing commonalities with the listener

- Finding ways to be different

- Using gestures and movement

- Using symbols and graphics

- Using metaphors and analogies

- Storytelling

- Using the environment

- Listening

- Asking the right questions

Let's take at look at each of these aspects within a leadership context.

Delivering the Message Clearly

Leaders must be able to order their thoughts, choose words that impart the message clearly, and be comfortable and at ease with the spoken word. Inarticulate leaders often feel self-conscious and are less likely to express their opinions and ideas or engage in conversations with followers. This greatly reduces their effectiveness and results in the loss of synergy between leader and follower.

The ability to express difficult or technical concepts in simple ways is essential if the message is going to be received. Some people believe that the larger and more complex the words a person uses, the more intellectual or important he or she sounds. Use of such language may be appropriate for presenting technical or highly complex information to a homogeneous, professional audience, but it does not apply when speaking to or with general audiences. Instead of the communication fostering a connection, the opposite happens: followers feel more distant from the leader. The gap widens, and followers focus on how they are different and perhaps less informed, less educated, or less intelligent than the leader.

This ability to express complex concepts simply is not always a natural talent. The good news is that it can be learned. At a department head meeting with approximately seventy managers attending, an executive of a six hundred–bed medical center gave a twenty-minute presentation on statistical tests of significance. These managers represented all hospital departments, and less than a handful had any formal research background. The speaker explained difficult, complex research concepts during the presentation in a way that everyone in the room could clearly understand. When one person asked this executive where and how she developed this ability, her response was interesting. In her graduate work, she had a professor who assigned a paper but left the choice of topic up to the student. Once the student selected the topic—quality, patient safety, teams, capitated care—she had to write the paper without ever using the word the paper was about. She explained how this taught her to find multiple ways of expressing the same concept. What a gift!

An easy, conversational style of communicating establishes rapport with receivers, whether in a large group or a smaller, more intimate gathering. Ideas flow more freely, and speakers and listeners are less reserved about expressing opinions and disagreements. Bennis (1989) believes that a good leader encourages dissent, establishing a climate that encourages expression of contrary ideas.

Body language congruent with the verbal communication substantiates the message sent. If the speaker uses words that ring with sincerity but makes limited eye contact, has a stiff posture, and makes reserved gestures, these lessen the impact of the message. When verbal and nonverbal messages contradict each other, the listener will have trouble interpreting the speaker's meaning. The receiver may leave the situation feeling baffled but unable to put a finger on what is wrong. The words sounded good, but some sense or intuition tells the listener that the sender did not really mean what he or she said. At one meeting, the agenda was to review and discuss recommendations from a project team. The leader and several members of the project team, all employees with the exception of one manager, were to present their recommendations to the executive team. The CEO started out by saying how important it was to have employees involved in these project teams because of their perspective and proximity to the work and problems being discussed. He also reaffirmed the executive team's commitment to having employees become more involved in major decisions that affected their work.

The team presented its findings while the executives listened politely. They asked a few questions and then graciously thanked and gently dismissed the project team members. Behind closed doors the real discussion began, and the executive team ended by discarding all the project team's recommendations. The executive team gave the following feedback to the project team: "Thanks for all your efforts," and "Your recommendations helped us clarify the issues and our thinking." Is it any wonder that members of the project team had mixed feelings—how to reconcile the courtesy and appreciation the executive team expressed with their feelings of exclusion and impotence?

Occasionally miscommunication is humorous, as the following story shows: "During his tenure as the director of the Federal Bureau of Investigation, J. Edgar Hoover once wrote in the margin of a draft letter: 'Watch the borders.' He intended only that his secretary widen the margins of the letter; what he got, due to a grand misinterpretation by some overzealous aides, was heightened readiness along the U.S.-Mexico border" (McDonald, 1997, p. 4). Of course, this story is funny only in retrospect. At the time it was a fairly costly miscommunication. Mixed messages can be dangerous because we often do not consciously recognize them. They leave us with vague feelings of discomfort but nothing that we can pin down or examine. Often they create a sense of discord, and although mixed messages may not lead immediately to a breakdown of trust, loss of trust is an eventual outcome.

The only foolproof way to determine the message's clarity is for the leader to seek feedback from the receiver. If the response is negative or if the receiver does not have clear enough understanding to act on the message, another attempt is in order. Ideally, through direct dialogue with the recipient, it may be possible to determine the source of confusion and clear it quickly. In any event, the communicator can resend the message, perhaps with additional information or a new explanation to increase clarity.

Creating a Message with Impact

Clear, concise information enhances the impact of messages. And an effective communicator knows how to emphasize the key points of a message by getting listeners' attention; establishing something in common with them; finding ways to be different; employing gestures and movement for key points; using metaphors and analogies; telling stories; employing symbols, graphics, audiovisuals, and the environment.

Gifted communicators use these methods effortlessly. Although some of these techniques are simpler and easier to use than others, all can become smooth with practice. Mastering these various methods is worth the effort because they will help the receiver to understand the message.

Getting the Listener's Attention

Gaining people's attention is an initial step in communicating. In formal presentations or discussions, a third party may introduce the communicator or the topic to the group. Most often listeners' eyes and minds focus on the leader because there is a natural beginning point. Just the presence of a known and admired leader may draw the attention of followers who are interested in communicating with him or her. In a few instances, however, the leader may need to specifically draw followers' attention in order to make a point. Effective ways of accomplishing this include using a hand gesture indicating the desire to speak or simply waiting for silence among the audience.

Establishing Commonalities with Listeners

Pointing out commonalities between the speaker and listeners is another way to gain attention and establish rapport or a sense of connection. This is difficult unless the leader knows something about the followers. The more familiarity the leader has with followers and their situation, the easier it is to identify common backgrounds, values, goals, and ideas. If the leader does not know a great deal about the followers, listening closely for free information is a useful strategy. This means being alert to information they share during conversations that may not pertain directly to the topic at hand but reveal something about the individuals in the group.

Dialogue between leader and follower often reveals many points of similarity. During the interchange of ideas, thoughts, and opinions or with the expression of concerns and fears, the leader who is in agreement with the follower, has had a comparable experience, or shares the follower's concerns or feelings can use these similarities. The leader may say something like: "Yes, I remember when I worked in the lab on the night shift, I often felt left out of the loop." Done briefly, without drawing attention away from the speaker, this establishes a commonality and sense of connection. Selected self-disclosure is a gift of trust that the leader extends to followers. Telling the listener "I know just how you feel" is detrimental because it sounds like a platitude or cliché. Some listeners may react with skepticism and anger if they do not believe that the person communicating understands. "When I was in a similar situation, I had some of the same feelings or reactions you are expressing" is a more realistic statement and communicates understanding without minimizing the uniqueness of the speaker's experience.

A dramatic example of this illustrates what happens when a leader emphasizes differences. Susan was the project director for a massive organizational initiative in a hospital in which she had been a nurse manager for years. She enlisted the services of an external consultant to assist with employee training. At the first session, she introduced herself, saying, "I am the hospital administrator in charge of this initiative." To this audience of nursing employees, the message was clear: Susan no longer considered herself a nurse. Many among them were taken aback. Susan's attempt to distance herself from her background was successful: she was so distant from these followers that she was ineffective in her new role.

Finding Ways to Be Different

Although it sounds contradictory to the point just made, being different is another way to emphasize a message. O'Dooley (1992, p. 7) writes, "People remember the unusual better than the ordinary." This can be as simple as a leader appearing informally instead of at preannounced, prearranged, and structured times; using overhead transparencies for a presentation instead of PowerPoint, or acting out a skit to demonstrate a major point. O'Dooley gives an example from his years selling photocopying machines for IBM, when he wanted customers to remember him over his competitors from Xerox and Kodak. He introduced himself as "Patrick O'Dooley, reproduction specialist." It worked in spite of the odd looks he received. "To stand out in others' minds, do things a little differently than everyone else does them."

When one large medical center undertook a massive restructuring project, the senior executive staff performed a skit to help deliver a message about the importance of the project and the role of employees. The skit included these executives in western garb, on horses, and revolved around a pioneer theme. The videotape of this skit was powerful—not just the overt message but the impact of seeing these leaders, in blue jeans and cowboy hats, on horses. It was dramatic.

Using Gestures and Movement

Accenting key points with gestures, movement, or tone of voice helps anchor the message for listeners. Useful in casual conversations as well as more formal discussions and presentations, movement draws the listener's attention and increases the likelihood that the listener will remember the point. Controlled hand and arm gestures can be used to communicate emphasis. Effusive, broad gestures may raise suspicion about the speaker's level of sincerity and should be avoided. Changing the tone or volume of voice can be effective. Either softening or increasing the volume causes the receiver to listen more closely.

Using Symbols and Graphics

Enhancing a message with symbols, graphics, and audiovisuals can increase its clarity. A good graphic display often communicates a message in a way that makes words unnecessary. The graphic has to be one the audience can understand, of course. Audiovisuals are useful adjuncts to formal presentations, and many sources, especially training journals and materials, can provide ideas for making them more effective. PowerPoint presentations can be an effective tool but may be overused. One health care system banned executives and leaders from using them because it caused competition among presenters. PowerPoint presentations had become glitzier and more technologically advanced until they totally distracted members of the audience from the message meant to be communicated.

Symbols are capable of motivating human behavior. They are very powerful and anything but benign. In an article about the use of symbols in health care, Clark (1996, p. 20) gives some evocative examples:

> A firefighter carries a lifeless toddler from the bomb scene at Oklahoma City's federal building. In the South Bronx, the athletic shoes of youths killed by violent means are hung from fire escapes and clotheslines. In New Mexico, crosses adorned with flowers mark the roadside where a loved one has been killed in an alcohol-related automobile accident. Mementos left at the Vietnam Veteran's Memorial. The homespun patchwork of the national AIDS quilt. Blouses tied together to signify the women who have been battered and killed as a result of domestic violence. Yellow ribbons as a remembrance of someone missing from home, red ribbons for those who died of AIDS, pink ribbons for the fight against breast cancer. . . . All these images represent the shared experience of Americans, with respect to our health and well-being.

With the passing years, the list of symbols can include even more contemporary images, such as the collapse of the World Trade Center or the images of a U.S. soldier holding an Iraqi prisoner by a leash.

The communication may use symbolic language or behavior without conscious intent or even awareness. Termination of employees or announcements of major decisions on Fridays may symbolically distance the sender from receivers of the message by the physical separation of the weekend. Executive offices far from the workers may be practical for executives wanting limited accessibility but create a daunting prospect for employees. The hierarchy often plays out consistently within the executive offices—the CEO is located farthest from the front door, buffered by layers of secretarial staff. In what ways does this symbolize the leader-follower relationship?

Using Metaphors and Analogies

Another way to increase impact is by using metaphors and analogies to help people relate their own experiences and understanding to the message. Metaphors are comparisons in which we describe something as if it were something else. Analogies involve a comparison between two cases or things and infer that what is true in one case is true in another. Songwriters and poets use metaphors and analogies extensively. So do effective leaders in health care organizations.

One hospital, which usually had eight labor and delivery rooms available, was undergoing major renovation in that department. The entire department seemed to be torn apart; at one particularly difficult time, desk drawers from the central nurses' station were placed on the floor down both sides of the hallway. With ten active labor patients in the department, there was absolute chaos. The leader remarked, "This is like having a dinner party for ten while your kitchen is being remodeled!" This humorous observation diffused some of the high emotion and created a picture in people's minds that helped them understand and appreciate their frustration.

Storytelling

Storytelling is one of the most effective tools a good communicator uses. There is magic in stories. Throughout history, people have relied on narration and storytelling to express ideas that are difficult to communicate any other way. Abraham Lincoln was a consummate storyteller and is a wonderful example of a leader who was able to use conversation, humor, and stories to make his point and convince listeners of his way of thinking. Phillips, in his fascinating book *Lincoln on Leadership* (1992, p. 157), writes: "Nearly everyone who came in contact with our sixteenth president heard him relate some kind of yarn. Lincoln, it turned out, had an overwhelming inventory of anecdotes, jokes, and stories; furthermore, he possessed the ability to instantly pull out just the right one for any situation that might arise. Lincoln was a master at the art of storytelling, and he used that ability purposefully and effectively when he was president of the United States."

The best storytellers collect ideas and anecdotes continually. They are always looking for examples that make a point or that they can use to illustrate a complex or emotional concept. And the excellent storyteller practices sharing the tale over and over again until it is convincing. The astute leader knows that successful organizations and teams are "storied" organizations and teams. They listen to the stories circulating and think about what these stories say about the culture. Do the stories reflect positive values and aspirations of the organization? Do they create enthusiasm and loyalty among followers?

In one urban tertiary medical center, the organization mission statement and values were beautifully inscribed, framed, and strategically mounted in every office and conference room of the facility. They described a wonderful organization—words with heartfelt meaning that anyone would aspire to reaching. Amazingly, the predominant flavor of stories circulating in the organization was exactly the opposite. The favorite stories, repeated with great fervor, highlighted personal and professional corruption of the executive staff, unscrupulous maneuvering of managers against peers and employees, and malicious whisperings suggesting various reasons for promotions. The stories revealed the organization's true culture. But stories do not have to be this extreme to have negative impact.

People remember stories longer than they can recall data and facts. Students of leadership theory and effectiveness confirm storytelling as a strategy and emphasize the role of stories "as powerful motivational tools that spread loyalty, commitment, and enthusiasm" (Phillips, 1992, p. 158). Peters and Austin (1985, pp. 278, 281) note that "human beings reason largely by means of stories, not by mounds of data. Stories are memorable. . . . They teach." A leader who understands this pays more attention to the role that stories and myths play in communicating ideals, values, and direction.

In a southern 280-bed hospital, a massive restructuring and work redesign initiative was under way. Teams were developed and functioning in many of the patient-care areas. During the most trying week for the newly implemented teams, the community experienced a serious flu epidemic, and the hospital census hit a peak. Employees had been stretched well beyond their capacity; tempers were short; and absenteeism due to the flu ensured that the upcoming weekend was going to be a calamity. On Saturday the vice president for patient-care services was pitching in and helping out on the patient-care units. One of the most pressing needs was cleaning the patients' bathrooms. People in the patient-care departments were captivated and heartened to hear the story of how this vice president rolled up her sleeves and began cleaning toilets. The story of this doctorally prepared nurse doing what most needed to be done for patients' comfort and cleanliness still circulates in this organization. People here understand the organization's values of "patients come first" and teamwork.

During the blizzard of 1996, many health care facilities in the Northeast generated stories that today tell new employees about the organization's culture. Executives in jeans and sweatshirts served food in the cafeteria to hungry staff; employees with four-wheel-drive vehicles transported colleagues to and from work; and countless other examples exemplified leadership and strong organizational values.

Perhaps some of the most poignant stories come from times of disaster such as the San Francisco earthquake of 1989, Hurricane Andrew in southern Florida, the Oklahoma City bombing, or 9/11. During these times of crisis, people rise to meet heartbreaking challenges, and leadership emerges. Rosemary Jacobson, then CEO of United Health Systems (now Altru Health System) in Grand Forks, North Dakota, describes in personal correspondence with the author (May 20, 1997) the disaster of the record-breaking 1997 spring flooding:

> During the early morning hours of Friday, April 18, the dikes within the city began to fail, forcing mandatory evacuations of several large neighborhoods in Grand Forks and East Grand Forks. The state health officer called me Friday evening and informed me that the water system and infrastructure would fail. I still believed we would be able to keep United dry and open.
>
> It took only a few hours for realization to set in. I knew we would not be able to manage care of 197 inpatients without water or sewer for an extended period of time. Because of this, the decision was made to evacuate all 197 hospital patients and 371 nursing and retirement home residents from Medical Park and the Grand Forks community. This was accomplished within a 24-hour period.
>
> Our evacuation could only have been accomplished with teamwork. We spent many, many hours planning the Altru Health System, and it paid off. We functioned as a team anyone would be proud to know.

This emergency evacuation was the largest hospital evacuation since Saigon fell to the Vietcong during the Vietnam War. Stories about disasters endured and calamities shared can strongly bond people together. These stories survive and serve to inspire and hearten, as well as to illustrate the basic beliefs and values of the people in the organization.

Using the Environment

Creative use of the environment is another powerful method of making a point. A good example is one clever speaker's presentation to a group of human resource specialists, executives, and trustees about the cost of discrimination when an organization does not solicit members of minorities for governing board positions. Knowing the audience would be approximately 98 percent male, the speaker had interspersed throughout the audience pairs of high heels in front of empty chairs—a visual reminder to this highly homogeneous audience of at least one underrepresented minority!

John, CEO of a major health care system, was having trouble with followers who were continually late to regular meetings. The group discussed punctuality as a team value repeatedly but to no avail. Finally, John decided to communicate the message differently. On the day of his next meeting with the system vice presidents, John went to the boardroom and locked the door as the meeting was scheduled to begin. Ten minutes later the first vice president arrived and was dismayed to find the door locked. Within twenty minutes all attendees were gathered outside the boardroom, where they waited anxiously until the scheduled meeting was over. When John finally opened the door, he told them that if they weren't on time, he would make decisions without them. News of that locked door spread like wildfire throughout the organization. The message was clear and communicated, simply through a locked door.

A different leader facing the same problem started her meetings on time regardless of whether anyone else had yet arrived. The impact of coming into a room to find the leader talking to herself, conducting the meeting with no participants, made a tremendous impression not just on the first follower to finally arrive but on everyone else who heard the story. People got the message.

Listening

A discussion of spoken communication would be incomplete without considering the skill of listening. As important as the ability to be articulate is the leader's ability to listen. "The common image of leaders is that they are great talkers, charismatic and articulate. Far more important is that they are great listeners" (Berry, 1992, p. 2). Giving attention to others' thoughts, ideas, and opinions allows a leader deeper understanding of the follower. Listening for emotions and feelings ensures that the leader understands a message fully, as these elements are difficult for many people to express verbally. Nothing is so powerful as a leader who has accurate facts and information and realizes that followers are an excellent source of both. Not only does it lead to better decision making, but it increases the shared meaning between leaders and followers. Other notable reasons for developing good listening skills are that the listener can learn new information, that listening provides time to digest ideas and fully attend to the entire message, and that listening communicates respect and caring to the speaker.

Listening Provides New Information

Exemplary listening skills enable the leader to learn and gather information not previously known. The comment "When you speak you only repeat what you already know; it is when you listen that you might learn something" has been attributed to Abraham Lincoln. Not listening to others conveys an attitude of arrogance, intended or not. They will perceive the nonlistener as not needing input from anyone else because the leader feels all-knowing and correct. Listening to others generates ideas, especially for meeting the resistance someone has to the leader's approach. New ideas blend with the leader's ideas and serve as a catalyst for a unique thought or strategy.

Listening Provides Time to Reflect

We can think faster (about three to four times) than words can be spoken. As you listen, think about what the person communicating is trying to say. Does the individual's body language match his or her words? Does the message fit previous experiences you have had with this individual? How does the speaker's message fit with previous thinking on this topic? Do the ideas expressed stir any other thoughts or possibilities?

Listening Communicates Caring

Listening to an individual express ideas and thoughts has a powerful impact on the speaker. Perhaps nothing else the leader can do communicates respect and caring for the follower as much as showing interest in what the follower has to say. M. Scott Peck, in *The Road Less Traveled* (1978, pp. 81, 120–121), defines *love* as "the will to extend one's self for the purpose of nurturing one's own or another's spiritual growth." He goes on to point out: "When we love another we give him or her our attention; we attend to that person's growth. . . . When we attend to someone, we are caring for that person. The act of attending requires that we make the effort to set aside our preoccupations and actively shift our consciousness. Attention is an act of will, of work against the inertia of our own minds. . . . By far the most common and important way in which we can exercise our attention is by listening."

Increasing Listening Skills

Communication courses often teach the skill of listening, and leaders with a background in a discipline that emphasizes and requires listening ability, such as counseling or social work, are at an advantage with this skill. The good news is that it is a personal skill and, as such, can be learned and improved with practice. It is common to overrate one's listening ability because it seems so simple. Peck (1978, p. 121) points out, "Listening well is an exercise of attention and by necessity hard work. It is because they do not realize this or because they are not willing to do the work that most people do not listen well."

The best leaders are great listeners. There are many helpful pointers they have learned as they worked at improving their listening skills:

- *Work at listening and continually attempt to increase your listening span.* Good listeners control any temptation to interrupt or draw attention away from the speaker. Some people grapple for the right words to express their ideas and may take longer to finish their thoughts. Interrupting them only extends this process and gives a speaker the clear message that the listener finds that what he or she is saying is not important enough to wait for its full expression. As Peck (1978) points out, our attention needs to be conscious.
- *Take the time to listen.* Not everyone is able to speak extemporaneously in a clear and concise manner. Instead they may think out loud and gradually grope their way to their meaning. Their first statement may be only a vague approximation of what they mean. For the speaker to open up and crystallize the meaning of a message, the listener must convey a feeling that there is plenty of time to speak freely. Some leaders rationalize that they are too busy to listen. A good leader is too busy *not* to listen. The leader who does not take time to listen may miss crucial information and never achieve needed understanding. A good listener makes mental or actual notes of items to remember.
- *Listen for understanding rather than to reply.* Stephen Covey (1990, p. 237) believes that the single most important principle he has learned in the field of interpersonal relations is to "seek first to understand, then to be understood." Instead of focusing on preparing a reply to the speaker or thinking about how to make himself or herself understood, the listener actively tries to understand what the speaker is saying. Sometimes by taking on the behaviors of being a good listener, we find that the act of listening may follow.

A good listener stays alert, establishes eye contact with the speaker, leans forward if appropriate, shows interest by nodding the head or raising the eyebrows, and encourages the speaker to continue by asking thoughtful and appropriate questions. Jane Fonda once said that putting on her exercise clothes puts her in the frame of mind to work out. In the same way, effective listeners who don effective listening behavior may find it leads to that very behavior.

• *Listen in spite of the delivery method.* Some speakers are more difficult to listen to than others. The speaker may have been blessed with wonderful ideas and thoughts but have a boring, monotone voice or a face without much expression. Good listeners aren't as concerned about mannerisms or delivery but focus on the message itself. They ask: What can I learn from this speaker? They know that not everyone is a brilliant, witty conversationalist.

• *Listen in spite of the content.* If the content of the message is one that evokes strong emotion in the listener, it can be very difficult to not respond emotionally and interrupt the speaker. The listener can become excited or upset, especially when what the speaker says ignites pet peeves or challenges personal convictions or prejudices. It is easy to judge the speaker's comments too hastily, and this can close down further communication.

• *Remove external distractions and resist internal distractions.* Distractions create noise in the system and make communication an even tougher job for both speaker and listener. If this is an especially important conversation, move the dialogue someplace where distractions are at a minimum, even if it means delaying it. A good listener recognizes and admits internal distractions and suggests alternate times for the speaker to return.

Participants at a national conference were taking a break in the middle of a three-hour session. The speaker had just discovered that she had left her purse in the rest room earlier that morning. As the speaker was leaving the conference room in a panic, a participant approached her and attempted to engage her in a discussion. The speaker listened politely for a moment and then explained her present inability to listen. She told the participant she would be back soon, when they could then talk. But the participant tried to continue the conversation, at which point the speaker said, "You don't understand. I cannot hear a word you're saying because I am upset about losing my purse. Let's talk when I return."

This is the same conversation a leader needs to have with a follower if the time just is not right to listen. With the emphasis on an open-door policy and total accessibility of the leader, it may seem contradictory to ask the person to come back at a better time. However, if distractions are just too great, it is better to be honest than to pretend and risk missing an important message. Of course, the listener must make certain that the follow-up conversation occurs.

• *Restate or paraphrase the message.* When the speaker is finished, the listener should restate what he or she heard and understood as the message. This is very affirming to the speaker and also allows the speaker to clarify, if the listener received an inaccurate message. This very powerful technique is often referred to as reflective listening because it reflects back to the speaker on major points of the message.

These suggestions can help increase listening effectiveness but probably even more important is that the leader-listener continually evaluates his or her level of listening ability. Is it improving? Do followers believe they have been heard and understood? How often are miscommunications occurring as a result of poor listening? In addition to using these principles, effective listeners understand that there are several levels of listening.

Levels of Listening

In *The Seven Habits of Highly Effective People* (1989), Stephen Covey identifies several different levels of listening. The lowest level is ignoring, when the person is not listening at all. This occurs when we tune someone or something out totally. Pretend listening is the second level, when the "listener" may nod and behave in a manner that suggests listening without hearing a word. The standard example of this is when one's spouse is reading the paper or watching a favorite sports event on television and distractedly responds to questions that he or she does not even hear. Selective listening is hearing only chosen parts of the conversation. The leader who is interested in agreement from followers may hear only positive elements of feedback and ignore or discount more unfavorable segments. The fourth level is attentive listening, in which the listener pays attention and focuses energy on the words being said. The fifth and highest level is empathic listening, which involves understanding not only the words of the message but its emotion and meaning.

Whether we call it active, reflective, or empathic listening, this is the only form of listening that focuses completely on the listener and puts the listener in the speaker's frame of reference. Its purpose is to fully comprehend what the speaker is expressing, and it goes even further by adding the feedback loop to give the speaker a response that reflects this understanding. The power of this communication technique is that it gives the speaker the opportunity to correct misperceptions or misunderstandings immediately. When a listener uses reflective or empathic listening, the speaker feels understood and validated.

Use of this technique requires the listener's judgment and skill. Reflecting back the speaker's words and perceived emotion is a direct invitation to the speaker to continue. If the listener does not have time to follow through fully, use of this technique may send a mixed message. Practice and refinement of this skill are necessary so that the listener is not just parroting the speaker's words (an irritating and foolish thing to do!). The listener may say something like: "Let me check this out. I thought I heard you say. . . ." "Are you saying . . . ?" "It sounds like you're feeling. . . . Am I right?" Until this is part of the listener's repertoire, it may feel uncomfortable, but the benefits are tremendous.

Using empathic listening helps a listener stay actively in the listening mode and focus solely on the speaker. If the listener has to repeat the essence of the message to the speaker, it focuses his or her attention tremendously. It puts the listener in the speaker's frame of reference and increases the listener's understanding of the speaker. Virtually no other technique is as helpful in building a solid relationship. The disadvantage is that the listener has no sense of control or efficiency. So although this method is effective, it may not feel efficient. It is efficient in the sense that it prevents miscommunications.

A signal to you that you are not using empathic listening occurs when someone conveys the same message repeatedly. The problem is that you may not have provided any feedback indicating that you received the message. An example of this occurred in a team of executives that had formed to attend a long-term learning program together. Members of the team were handpicked and were required to commit to attending a series of four three-day sessions over a year. As part of the selection criteria, all agreed that they would attend every session. After two sessions Cal told his other team members that he would be missing the next session. His team members were justifiably angry and gave him that feedback. One member, Jill, told him directly that she felt he was letting the team down and she was very disappointed in him. He showed no response.

In another week the team met again to discuss what they would do with Cal's decision to miss the next three-day session. Again Jill gave Cal the same feedback, and he showed no response. The team was having difficulty dealing with this dilemma and met one last time to decide whether Cal should remain on the team after the missed session. Again the teammates expressed their concern and anger, with Jill again directly telling Cal how she felt. Cal became very angry in return and said to Jill, "You've said that three times now; will you stop beating a dead horse? I'm getting tired of hearing this." Jill was surprised and replied, "I didn't think you ever heard me because you showed no response."

Followers who believe they have not been heard do one of two things. They may stop trying, believing that the leader does not care or is not interested in their opinions or ideas. If they are more persistent, however, they may continue to repeat a message until the leader acknowledges it. To be effective listeners, good leaders pay attention; and if they are hearing the same message repeatedly, they ask themselves: "Why am I hearing this again? Have I acknowledged this message?"

Listening is a skill that takes time to develop and continual attention to keep improving. The payoff is tremendous. One of the most remarkable benefits of listening to others is that it becomes reciprocal. If leaders want to increase the probability that others will listen to what they have to say, they will start listening (Campbell and Inguagiato, 1994).

Asking the Right Questions

Few people consider asking questions an art form, and yet asking questions requires a much higher level of skill than most people think. The leader can use questions to gain information, obtain a different point of view, show respect for followers, and make them feel important and valued. And there is another benefit (Oakley and Krug, 1993, p. 150): "Smart communicators ask questions not only so they can hear the answers, but so the person asked can hear their own answers and thereby gain clarity for themselves or internalize something they have grasped only intellectually." Oakley and Krug go on to describe questions as a gift to the person being asked, just as answers are a gift to the asker.

Tips for more powerful questioning techniques that can increase the skill of the individual asking the questions include the following:

- *State the reason for the question.* Letting the person know why you are asking the question can eliminate resistance or the feeling of unwarranted curiosity. "Help me understand this better," or "I would like to understand the factors you considered when you made this decision."
- *Make it enjoyable for the other person.* Be enthusiastic and the person being questioned will feel positive.

- *Show interest in what the other person is saying.* Through body language, show an attentive attitude. This includes good eye contact, nodding or tilting the head, and appropriate facial expressions.
- *Use open-ended rather than closed questions.* Closed questions can be answered with a yes, no, or other one-word answer, which does not provide the breadth of communication the asker desires. It is the difference between saying: "Do I have your support on this project?" versus "What parts of this project can you support? What elements will you have difficulty supporting?"
- *Avoid creating the feeling of the third degree.* Giving followers the third degree puts them on the defensive, even if they were feeling open in the beginning. One question after another delivered in a rapid-fire manner is certain to elicit a negative reaction in most people.
- *Ask for their opinion.* A very powerful question is one that simply solicits the person's thoughts about a particular issue or situation: "What do you think about . . . ?" Of course, the person asking the question has to be truly interested or risks sending a mixed message.
- *Repeat key words from answers and summarize thoughts.* This indicates to the person responding to the questions that you have listened to and heard him or her.
- *Share appreciation of responses.* Let the speakers know that you appreciate their thoughts and the time they have given to answer your questions. "Thank you for going through this with me so that I can understand it better."

Sometimes leaders are afraid that if they seek opinions from others and listen carefully to their answers and ideas, this communicates implicit agreement with these ideas. This is one reason feedback to the speaker is important. It is possible to listen attentively and yet clearly tell the individual when there is disagreement on an idea. Good questioners continually monitor other people's reactions to their questioning techniques. Does their technique facilitate the flow

of information? Do people open up more, or are they becoming qui-
eter and more reserved? This feedback gives the questioner direct
information on the effectiveness of his or her technique.

Nonverbal Communication

Intertwined closely with spoken communication is nonverbal communication. Sometimes referred to as body language, *nonverbal
communication* is actually a broader term and can include the use of
time, space, and the environment as well. Verbal and nonverbal
messages must match, or they create confusion and frustration. Of
these two channels of communication, nonverbal language can be
more potent, as demonstrated by the childhood game of Simon
Says. Simon gives rapid oral instructions while demonstrating the
requested behavior. Participants follow the leader's movements, and
the unlucky players who continue to follow the leader even in the
absence of the phrase "Simon says" lose the game. The point is that
people are more likely to emulate behavior than to follow words or
directives.

The potential power of nonverbal language compels the effective leader to observe and understand the significance of certain
body language and to continually examine his or her own nonverbal communication for the messages it sends. Leaders who are sensitive to these messages have greater control over their ability to
communicate with clarity. In the same way, a leader becomes more
skilled at interpreting others' messages by tuning in to nonverbal
cues. Important nonverbal messages can be conveyed through the
following:

- Use of time

- Touch

- Use of space

- Appearance

- Body motions and posture

- Choice of words and voice tone

- Eye behavior

Use of Time

The leader's use of time communicates a clear message about what the leader believes is important. This relates back to the concept of visibility and accessibility in the discussion of trust. Are followers able to reach the leader? Is there time to dialogue on important issues and concerns? With whom does the leader spend the most time? Who doesn't get any of the leader's time? Allowing enough time in a busy schedule to periodically have coffee or lunch with followers is a practical way of keeping in touch with what is happening. This can be difficult for more introverted leaders for whom casual, spontaneous conversation does not come easily. Sometimes scheduled, structured meeting times, even though the meeting itself is informal, can ease the way for this leader.

Touch

In this country the issue of touch is more complex because of the increased focus on sexual harassment. Anything that could be construed to be intimate or sexual is unacceptable. Even if it doesn't result in litigation, it leads to distrust between leader and follower. Casual contact can actually improve the relationship because it connotes acceptance and caring. A famous classic research study involved a librarian who was asked to lightly and impersonally touch students on the arm when the librarian checked out books to them or answered their questions. The students in the experimental group whom the librarian touched rated the librarian as more helpful, intelligent, and personable than did the students in the control group. The librarian was the same individual and otherwise treated the students identically.

Other cultural differences influence the use of touch (Morris, 1979). North Americans and northern Europeans have noncontact cultures, which means that body contact and touch are not common except in prescribed arenas. Arabs and Latins, however, are high-contact people and would consider North Americans and northern Europeans reserved, cool, and downright uptight. Family differences can also account for touch being more or less acceptable. Some people come from affectionate, demonstrative families where hugging is common. Other people are uncomfortable with hugging even in social situations because they reserve this behavior for their intimates. Paying close attention to a follower's reaction to touch alerts the leader to its appropriateness.

Use of Space

Both space and spacing are issues to consider when evaluating nonverbal messages. Space can connote status: the person with the best and most space usually has the highest status. A corner office with windows is often touted as the highest-status executive space. The size and location of the work space send a message indicating value and worth. Does the organization allot space for classrooms and adequate room for employee lounges? Is there a special physician dining room? Is there reserved parking for executives and managers? In the same way, reserved parking for an employee of the month indicates value and esteem. What messages are the organization's leadership sending?

Another issue related to space is that of territoriality (Morris, 1979). Humans are highly territorial, and this translates to an inherent compulsion to possess and defend space that they perceive as their property. Participants at a meeting or a conference choose a chair and put up boundaries to indicate to others where their space begins and ends. A coat on the chair, a notebook and coffee cup strategically placed all indicate possession of space. Employees carve out their space in the workplace and may then feel violated if they return to find someone else in "their" chair, at "their" desk, using "their" telephone or computer.

Respect for an individual's space is an important issue because organizations often show a complete lack of regard or concern for an employee's space, especially frontline employees. Departments are relocated, offices moved, and space invaded, often without any acknowledgment of the impact on the individual. To build trust between leaders and followers, each must show care and respect for the other's work and personal spaces.

Personal space is another concept the excellent communicator understands. North American adults who are interacting in a professional or business capacity generally have four basic and distinct distances of interaction (Morris, 1979):

1. Intimate zone: ranging from actual physical contact to about two feet
2. Personal zone: ranging from about two to four feet
3. Social zone: extending from about four to twelve feet
4. Public zone: stretching from twelve feet to the limits of hearing and sight

If someone violates an individual's space by coming too close, the result is increased tension and distrust. Common cues are that the individual reduces eye contact, moves away, or puts something (like a chair, table, or desk) between him- or herself and the speaker. Leader-follower relationships usually begin in the social zone, and after trust has been established, they move into the personal zone.

Seating arrangements at a meeting send a message. When the leader joins others in the break room for a cup of coffee and always chooses to sit at the head of the table, it may send a message that he or she expects always to be in charge. In a formal meeting, with several people around the table, sitting straight across from someone who holds an adversarial position tends to increase conflict between the two parties. Sitting next to each other reduces the amount of conflict. A too-crowded conference or meeting room can increase hostility. Power is also ascribed to the person on whose turf the meeting is taking place. Does the leader go to where followers are, or do followers always come to the leader? Especially in resolving conflict, the leader can equalize power by using a neutral territory.

Appearance

An individual's dress and appearance send a message to others. Like it or not, physical appearance makes an impression on others within the first five to seven seconds of contact. Although this is not about dressing for success or impressing your followers, it is a reminder to consider the importance of the leader-follower relationship and the need to establish rapport and trust with those followers. Rapport is built by others perceiving sameness rather than difference. If the leader is trying to impress those higher in the hierarchy, the old dress-for-success model is appropriate. Peers or those who are lower in the hierarchy are more often impressed when they can see what they have in common with the leader. Some of these issues become clouded when formal hierarchy is part of the leader-follower relationship. A peer- or employee-leader is more likely to dress like the followers. If followers are in scrub clothes and uniforms, a leader in a navy blue business suit may inadvertently emphasize differences. On the other hand, if an employee-leader normally wears scrub clothes to work and is now leading an interdisciplinary task force that is more formal, showing up in scrub clothes may reduce the leader's effectiveness.

Body Motions and Posture

Body motions and posture send distinct messages. Posture and gestures clearly communicate passive, aggressive, and assertive behaviors. Slumped posture indicates passive behavior. Restricting hand and arm movement, hiding the hands, gripping one arm with the opposite hand, and holding hands rigidly at the side reinforce an impression of a nonassertive individual. Clenched teeth suggest aggressive behavior, as do a jaw jutted forward, tight lips, flushed cheeks, flared nostrils, a thrusting arm with a pointed index finger, pounding of fists, hands on hips, or clenched fists. The assertive leader uses more moderate and less frequent facial movement that expresses emotion congruent with the communication. Hand and arm movements are fluid, with hands held open and in view.

Leaders who sit in relaxed positions are able to influence followers better, and followers will see them as more persuasive and active. They are generally better liked than those who sit tightly and in a closed manner with arms crossed and held across the chest. Standing over others is seen as dominance; although it is appropriate in some settings (giving a formal speech), it would be too intimidating in others (at an informal or spontaneous meeting).

Some gestures are considered universal signals: hands over the head for surrender, saluting, shrugging the shoulders, and blowing a kiss. However, leaders who understand cultural differences are aware of the importance of accurately assessing the followers' body language; otherwise signals from one culture may lead to misinterpretation by followers in another. Every culture has its own body language, and children learn these nuances as they grow up. A North American who had traveled in Japan related this story: he and his wife were very impressed with the politeness of the Japanese schoolchildren who would stand by the side of the road and wave at cars going past. On their third day, they commented to the hotel desk clerk about how polite the children were. Imagine their chagrin when he told them that Japanese children stand at the side of the road and wave to indicate that they want to cross the street! They had totally misinterpreted this behavior.

Leaders need to understand the significance of their followers' cultural behaviors. In Japan, for example, workers despise being surprised at meetings. Each worker-follower expects the leader to take him or her aside privately to deliver word of any upcoming changes.

The ramifications for the leader are significant. Anticipating and understanding cultural differences allow a leader to communicate more effectively. People do not hear the intended message if they are embarrassed, insulted, or intimidated. This represents a tremendous challenge in today's multicultural and diverse ethnic environment.

Choice of Words and Voice Tone

This chapter has explored the effect of metaphors and use of language to evoke meaning. Health care is liberally sprinkled with military metaphors (Annas, 1996). People talk of *doing battle* with disease; patients are given *shots* or endure *invasive* procedures; and employees *on duty* are *in uniform*. In emergency departments patients are *triaged*, and surgery takes place in the *operating theater*. "When we use language like this, the force of the metaphor powerfully conveys our values, past experiences, and what we consider legitimate. . . . The truth lurks in the metaphor" (Henry and LeClair, 1987, p. 23). For this reason, leaders need to be very careful about the words they use. Referring to unconscious patients as *vegetables*, to people who cannot pay their bill as *write-offs*, to employees as *bodies*, FTEs (full-time equivalents), and *drones* communicates the way the leader values people. One health care manager was well known in her organization for joking about wanting to "lobotomize" employees so that they would be more compliant. Even though this conversation almost always occurred behind closed doors, it certainly affected her leadership ability and reflected how she valued people.

Voice tone and volume also communicate congruence or discrepancy with the words being said. An assertive tone of voice is usually one that has moderate volume and emphasis on words, a tone of voice appropriate for one adult speaking with a peer. Aggression is communicated with a loud voice, a heavy emphasis on certain words, and a parental tone. Nonassertive, or passive, voice is usually a soft, perhaps inaudible monotone or a childlike delivery.

Eye Behavior

Eye contact is culturally determined. North Americans are very careful about how and when they meet another person's eyes. An honest person looks another straight in the eye; shifty eyes connote dishonesty. North Americans avoid eye contact when walking down the street in a large city, when they are uncomfortable, or sometimes when they ask a question. In contrast, Israelis stare at each other on the street, not breaking eye contact until they have passed each other. In many Eastern cultures, direct eye contact is considered impolite. In England polite listeners will fix the speaker with an attentive stare and blink their eyes periodically as a sign of interest.

Direct eye contact in North America is considered assertive, usually meaning the individual is comfortable with looking another straight in the eye. Too piercing a stare can be intimidating, and narrowing the eyes is often considered aggressive. Eyes flitting back and forth between objects can give an individual the scared-rabbit look. Not looking a person directly in the eye causes the listener to wonder what the speaker is hiding.

Understanding the nuances of nonverbal communication not only enables the effective communicator to transmit clearer, more congruent messages but also assists both the speaker and listener in interpreting the signals they read. This process often occurs in retrospect, after miscommunication has occurred. Continually evaluating the effectiveness of one's communication leads to better results later.

Written Communication

Studies reveal that leaders who hold managerial or executive positions spend approximately three-quarters of their day in spoken communication with others (Mintzberg, 1980). But ideas are not exchanged exclusively by word of mouth. Although oral communication skills are more often used, writing skills are just as pivotal in a leadership practice. The ability to choose words carefully, express thoughts in writing, and create a document that helps followers understand a message leads to better communication. Clear and confident expression of the written word is an asset for any leader.

Of the three methods of communication—spoken, nonverbal, and written—the written form is most troublesome, if only because of its formal nature. "It is received cold, without the communicator's tone of voice or gesture to help. It is rigid; it cannot be adjusted to the recipients' reactions as it is being delivered. It stays 'on the record,' and cannot be undone. Further, the reason it is in fact committed to paper is usually that its subject is considered too crucial or significant to be entrusted to casual, short-lived verbal form" (Fielden, 1981, p. 42). For these reasons, a strong leader needs to be able to communicate effectively through writing.

The written word can be used to emphasize the importance of a message and serve as a record for future reference. Some people are visually oriented and prefer to see the message in writing to anchor it more solidly in their minds. Leaders today can write memos, letters, announcements, bulletins, newsletters, reports, and e-mail. The purpose and importance of the message determine which means to use. Because retrieving the written word once it is published is impossible, important written messages require a lot of thought and consideration. Considered one of the best leader-communicators of all time, Abraham Lincoln not only wrote his own speeches but was an eloquent public speaker and wrote "thousands of letters and notes to anyone with whom he felt he needed to communicate" (Phillips, 1992, p. 145). He believed in thorough preparation, often writing his thoughts over a long time and refining them later. This is still good advice today.

Important messages deserve the necessary time to ensure that they are well written and communicate the desired meaning. Being overly cautious, however, can result in an unreasonably prolonged communication process. In one organization, the executive team decided that it needed to write a letter to communicate with employees about several significant upcoming changes. The members of the team were so worried about litigation that various attorneys and team members took months to review the document, which then appeared so late that it was virtually useless. In addition, most of the intended audience could not understand what it really said. Remember to balance the need for accuracy, clarity, and caution.

E-mail

A relatively new method of written communication, e-mail has revolutionized the way we communicate. It has many advantages, including speed and ease of sending information. It enables closer and more timely contact between leaders and followers because it allows direct access to the leader.

On the downside, e-mail has replaced face-to-face communication in some organizations precisely because it is so easy. As with any written communication, a major disadvantage is that there is no tone of voice or body language to help the receiver interpret a message; and miscues can be serious. Tap out a message, hit the send key, and it is gone! This spontaneity has some disadvantages because it provides less thinking time. The final disadvantage of e-mail is also one of its benefits: it leaves no paper trail. Follow-up is more difficult to remember and yet more critical. Ross Perot's advice is to be cautious of using e-mail: "Treat e-mail like you would a snake. Don't let anybody communicate with you by e-mail. Have people come in and talk to you face to face, eyeball to eyeball" (Perot, 1996, p. 7). Although this may seem like extreme advice in this day and age, it is worth considering. Too many people today depend solely on e-mail for communication and neglect to realize the importance of emotional intelligence and the effect of face-to-face interaction in communication between leaders and followers. The emotionally intelligent leader realizes that it is important to be present and observe the other person's response to the message, to make adjustments spontaneously, using the listener's feedback cues to increase the flow and accuracy of information. This is difficult to impossible to do as well with e-mail.

Another disadvantage that also applies to the use of cellular phones and voice messaging is that we are just beginning to develop etiquette for these newer forms of communication. Until this etiquette becomes common practice, some people will unintentionally damage communication through these newer technologies rather than enhance it, such as by misusing e-mail to communicate difficult messages better transmitted face-to-face, by leaving lengthy voice mail messages with numbers and details that are difficult to capture in a message, by rambling on and on and producing quite lengthy e-mail messages, by blanketing the entire organization with e-mail messages that only a few individuals really need, by ignoring rules of grammar and courtesy because it is e-mail, and so on.

Improving Writing Skills

Fielden (1981, p. 42) identifies four categories to consider when writing:

- Readability

- Correctness

- Appropriateness

- Thought

The relative importance of each of these categories differs with the writer and situation, but considering each will increase a writer's effectiveness.

Readability

Readability depends on a clear style of writing. The leader needs to know the audience for whom he or she is writing in order to write clearly. The more general the audience, the simpler the sentences, and the less use of jargon, or shoptalk, the more readable the document. Liberal use of paragraphs, each beginning with a topic sentence, makes it easier for readers to grasp content quickly. Using simple language increases their comprehension of the material.

Another aspect of readability that Fielden (1981) identifies is the ability to lead the reader in an intended direction. The effective writer develops a skeleton structure first, to later flesh out with descriptive words. Clearly identifying the purpose and using transition sentences between paragraphs increase readability. Staying focused on the communication's main points takes less effort if the writer has clearly thought through what needs to be said.

Correctness

Correctness is a second category to consider when writing. This refers to much more than grammar and punctuation. Coherence and the ability to correctly position sentences and paragraphs increase the smoothness of the communication. Sentences logically flowing from one to another result in clearer understanding. An easy way to evaluate coherence is to ask someone with no knowledge of the topic or situation to review the document and give feedback.

Appropriateness

The third category, appropriateness, is related to how the writer presents the content. A leader writing a memo or announcement of a major initiative must first clarify in his or her own mind the communication's intent. Diplomacy is important: the reader who finds the tone of the document insulting or condescending will less easily accept the message. Giving enough information and using straight talk is better than employing flowery, convoluted language that passes for communication but is really just semantics.

Thought

Thought content of the communication is the last category to consider when writing. Content must be accurate and well organized. "Much disorganized writing results from insufficient preparation, from a failure to think through and isolate the purpose and the aim of the writing job. Most writers tend to think as they write; in fact, most of us do not even know what it is we think until we have actually written it down" (Fielden, 1981, p. 46). A carefully considered outline is of tremendous value to producing logical, well-presented information.

Careful analysis, bias-free evidence, and identification of working assumptions are all components of the written communication's content. If facts are part of the document, the document must carefully analyze them; and these facts must support the conclusions it draws. The writer may experience a tendency to state a conclusion without sharing any of the relevant facts with the reader, perhaps fearing that the reader would not draw the same conclusion. Supporting evidence that is logical and clearly presented serves to guide the reader in the direction that the writer seeks. The writer can share opinions if he or she identifies them as such and does not consider them hard evidence for a particular argument.

It is also the writer's responsibility to succinctly state any assumptions that are operating in the situation. This gives the reader the opportunity to agree or disagree with the assumptions and prevents potential disagreements with the actual content. A curriculum team was asked to develop a proposal for meeting employees' education needs during a planned cultural change in their system. When they presented the proposal, one of the first sections included the assumptions under which the team worked:

> People will not make cultural changes without new learning.
>
> Becoming something different is as important a goal as dealing with day-to-day issues.
>
> Leaders must model the desired behaviors.
>
> Expectations of employees must be clearly communicated and understood.

The investment in employee education is an investment in the future.

The most cost-effective approach must be found.

Simply identifying these assumptions generated tremendous dialogue with the executive team. As they talked through each assumption and examined the current reality of their system, they achieved an increased clarity of issues and needs. Both groups became more realistic about what the project could achieve.

Leaders communicating through written words need to avoid an effusive "con man" presentation meant to manipulate others. Simple words that ring with conviction and enthusiasm for an idea and for understanding the reader's point of view go further to convince readers of important points than an excess of flowery language. Keeping readability, correctness, appropriateness, and thought content foremost results in clearer written communication.

Summary

Effective communicators are skilled and versatile in all three modes of communication: spoken, nonverbal, and written. The leader must judge each situation to determine the appropriate means of sending a message and continually scan the outcomes of every communication to evaluate the effectiveness of the message transfer. Exemplary leaders know that the highest impact of message delivery occurs when the message is congruent among all three modes.

Special Communication Issues

Today's leader faces many challenges in attempting to communicate with clarity to all followers who need information:

- Communicating during change

- Communicating across geographical separations

- Communicating with teams

Communicating During Change

Health care is undergoing tremendous changes, in some instances almost cataclysmic in nature. The basic principles and techniques of good communication become even more important during times of rapid change because people seem to have an almost insatiable need for information at these times. Principles especially applicable during change include the following:

Be available and accessible.

Find multiple ways of describing a concept.

Articulate complex concepts as simply as possible.

Repeat key messages at least seven to nine times.

Share stories that communicate desired key values.

Make certain that the metaphors you use fit what you need to communicate.

Scrupulously avoid mixed messages—they are deadly in times of change.

Ask for feedback to ensure the message was received.

Remember that people are in a state of high emotion, which creates noise in their systems.

Separate resistance from learning and seeking information.

In addition to these principles, a key strategy during change is to develop specific communication approaches for key stakeholders. In *The Empowered Manager* (1987), Peter Block does a beautiful job of describing this strategy. He points out that a stakeholder is anyone who is needed for the success of the project or who can influence the project significantly. The first step is to identify the issue or change project and any key stakeholders whom this initiative will affect. The next step is to assess the stakeholders by the degree to which they agree with the project and the level to which they are trusted. The leader should not assume that a stakeholder agrees with the project. If the leader does not know the stakeholder's level of agreement, evaluation occurs after the leader sits down with the stakeholder and talks about the vision, purpose, or goals of the project or endeavor. This dialogue helps confirm or deny the stakeholder's agreement.

The leader then determines where the stakeholder fits into a specific matrix (Figure 4.2), depending on the level of trust in and agreement by the individual, both of which influence the communication strategy and effectiveness of message transfer. Opponents differ from adversaries only in the area of trust, but this difference dramatically affects the selection of communication strategies for each. A strategy for working with opponents is to keep communication lines open and to engage in frank and honest dialogue with them. Opponents are important because they value and trust the leader; they just do not agree with this particular initiative. With adversaries, however, there is not only a lack of agreement but a lack of trust. Dialogue is not particularly helpful because the leader

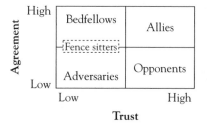

Figure 4.2. The Stakeholder Matrix

Source: The Empowered Manager by Peter Block, © 1987. Reprinted with permission of John Wiley & Sons, Inc., Hoboken, N.J.

Table 4.1. Strategies for Categories of Key Stakeholders

Allies

- Treat them as "one of us."

- Ask them honestly what they believe and see happening; listen to what they tell you.

- Continually discuss the project, vision, plan, and so on.

- Reaffirm the quality and importance of the relationship, especially that you appreciate their honesty.

- Acknowledge the doubts and vulnerability you feel.

- Ask for advice and support.

- Have regular meetings and ask them how they perceive things are going and what they need.

Opponents

- Reaffirm the quality of the relationship and the fact that it is based on trust.

- State your position; keep communication lines open.

- State in a neutral way what you think their position is.

- Engage in some kind of mutual problem solving.

Bedfellows

- Reaffirm any agreements.

- Acknowledge the caution that exists.

- Be clear about what you want from them in terms of working together and ask them to do the same.

- Try to reach some agreement on how you will work together.

Table 4.1. Strategies for Categories of Key Stakeholders, *continued*

Fence Sitters

- State your position.

- Ask where they stand, encourage them to express their opinion without judging them.

- Apply gentle pressure.

- Encourage them to think about the issue and let you know what it would take to give you their support.

Adversaries

- State your vision for the project.

- State in a neutral way your best understanding of your adversary's position.

- Identify your contribution to the problem.

- End the meeting with your plans and no demands.

Source: The Empowered Manager by Peter Block, © 1987. Reprinted with permission of John Wiley & Sons, Inc., Hoboken, N.J.

does not believe the adversary will be honest. Leaders using this model should be aware of a common error in judgment. This error occurs when a leader assumes that anyone who disagrees is an adversary. If the leader treats opponents like adversaries, they may in fact convert to this less desirable category. This happens when a supposed leader sees opposition as negative and all resisters as untrustworthy. A summary of appropriate strategies for each category is provided in Table 4.1.

Some difficulties are inherent in using this dynamic—not static—model. Through ongoing interchanges with stakeholders, continual reassessment both of their status on the matrix and of the effectiveness of a particular communication strategy selected is critical. Something in the environment or within the individual may have changed that alters his or her placement on the matrix. One manager whose organization was converting to a team-based structure was resistant to the idea of employee teams in his department, the business office. The leader identified him as an opponent according to Block's matrix (1987). His daughter visited over the holidays and told him about her experiences with employee work teams at her bank. She was enthusiastic, and after that weekend he was an ally! All it really took were concrete examples from a similar business, and he could see the possibilities. It also helped that he trusted his daughter explicitly and that she had no ulterior motives for trying to influence his opinion in this case.

A second drawback relates to accurately identifying where the stakeholder fits on the matrix. Some groups of stakeholders are so large that it is difficult to determine where each individual falls. To use this model, the leader must be able to dialogue directly with each stakeholder to determine agreement and choose a communication strategy based on this knowledge.

A cardiopulmonary leadership team in one organization used this model successfully for communicating with key physician stakeholders during a massive change initiative in their service center. The team consisted of the executive leader and the managers reporting directly to her. First, the team identified all key physician stakeholders and placed each on the matrix. In one or two instances, no one had enough information to make an accurate determination, so the team assigned each of those physicians to a team member. The team member's responsibility was to engage in a dialogue with the physician to determine that physician's understanding of the change being planned and level of support.

Once the team located all the physician stakeholders on the matrix, the team determined an appropriate communication strategy based on levels of trust and agreement for each. The team assigned all key stakeholders to a member of the leadership team to provide primary communication regarding this change initiative. This spread the responsibility of physician communication among all team members and allowed for a more individualized strategy for each stakeholder. The team implemented this project with greater support from more physicians than this team had previously experienced.

Communicating Across Geographical Separation

Today's leader has a new challenge: leading people from afar. Recent mergers, acquisitions, and consolidations of health care facilities have resulted in fewer stand-alone organizations (Blouin and Brent, 1997). With each passing year, the likelihood of geographically distant leaders increases. Leaders are managing and directing projects with representatives from multiple sites, which may or may not be within the community; more executives and managers today have responsibility for multiple facilities and departments; and the ascent of the virtual office coupled with the dejobbing of health care all combine to create the need for leaders who are effective in spite of geographical distance from their followers.

Geographical distance from followers creates significant barriers to applying any of the interpersonal competencies. Forming and nurturing a quality relationship can be difficult if two people are not physically proximate at least periodically. Dialogue over a computer or telephone line is not the same as face-to-face interaction. Distance makes communication more difficult and complicated. Just as the price for making a long-distance telephone call is higher than for a local call, so is the price exacted in a relationship when conducted long-distance. Pinchot and Pinchot (1996a, p. 18) articulate this issue very well: "As organizations become more complex, more geographically distributed, it becomes harder to create enough common vision and community spirit to guide the actions without increasing reliance on the chains of command. When people are separated by distance, vast differences in power and wealth, and conflict over resources and promotions, political struggle often replaces community. As the power of community is stretched thin, the chain of command becomes more prominent, and sense of community declines further."

The savvy leader applies the basic principles of communication and pays special attention to them when distance complicates the situation. In *Knights of the TeleRound Table* (1994), Kostner shares insights for executives who must manage from afar. Many of the principles she identifies are equally applicable to long-distance leaders. She points out that "the key way to build high performance across distance . . . is to build trust. Be obvious that every word, every action, every initiative on the virtual team builds trust" (p. 169). The paradox is that in these long-distance relationships, trust is more difficult to build but is even more important.

Other especially important principles in long-distance leader-follower relationships include the following:

Use strong symbols as a way of uniting people who are not in the same workplace.

Establish ways to help people learn more about each other so that they collaborate even when distant, such as on-site visits, kickoff meetings for key projects, and teleconferencing.

Use technology to link people across distances (a computer network, e-mail, and teleconferencing).

"Be scrupulously fair in treating all team members, near and far, equally. Even appearances or suggestions of favoritism break trust" (Kostner, 1994, p. 171).

Rely equally on followers whether on- or off-site (there is often temptation to rely more fully on those sharing the same geographical location).

Expect high performance equally from followers, not allowing distance to impede dealing with performance issues.

Leading from a distance is a growing challenge in today's workforce. We cannot overstate the importance of good communication. "Miscommunication, inequities of information, and unequal access to information are significant trust-breakers. . . . The impact of these remote problems may not show up for months, but will always negatively impact productivity and profits across distance" (Kostner, 1994, p. 172). Continually flowing communication and diligent sharing of information can counteract the out-of-sight, out-of-mind syndrome.

Communicating with Teams

In organizations that have converted to a team structure in their departments, leaders face the challenge of communicating with teams in addition to communicating with individuals or work groups. In each situation, the leader must be sensitive to the question: Is this an individual issue or a team issue? If it is a team issue, the leader must decide carefully how to communicate and with whom. Executives especially need to be careful about not usurping the team's responsibility and authority. There is often a strong tendency to access previous lines of communication and simply pick up the telephone and contact the manager to whom the team is responsible. Most managers willingly follow up and attain information or take the action the leader requested. Results are speedier and seem to simplify communication. However, the team may end up resenting the fact that the manager intervened in what the team members consider their work. An astute manager may put the leader directly in touch with the team so that the communication is as direct as possible.

When working with a group of individuals who have been selected as team representatives, a good leader makes certain they are clear about their role. Too often team members participate on ad hoc problem-solving teams or committees within the organization and forget that their role is to represent all of their teammates' interests and ideas. A simple reminder at each meeting helps these people focus on their need to return to their team and communicate with their colleagues. When the group discusses issues, asking attendees about their teammates' thoughts and ideas also reinforces their roles as team representatives.

Communicating with teams can complicate matters in an organization. The increased feeling of ownership and responsibility, as well as the improved outcomes that teams attain, usually outweighs the difficulties. However, there is a strong tendency for leaders to want to simplify reporting and communication relationships and to stay with the methods they have used in the past. A vivid example of this took place in a large medical center that was four years into the process of converting to a team-based structure. Employees in the risk management department had begun working together as a team. They were cross trained, self-directed, and self-managing. The director, Sammie, had been asked to investigate a particular problem, and she had turned the project over to the team.

These highly seasoned team members investigated the issue thoroughly and produced an outstanding report. Each proudly signed the work and asked to present it to the executive team. The executive team declined the team's request to present the report and instead asked Sammie to do the honors. Then, unbelievably, the executive team refused to accept the report with the team's signatures and insisted on the department director's signature only. Their reasoning was that the department director was solely accountable in case of any future problems. This demoralizing blow to an excited, enthusiastic, fully engaged team was devastating. It created a tremendous ripple of distrust and cynicism throughout the organization that these executive leaders never recognized. Employees in this organization no longer believed that executive leaders understood what it meant to be on a team. And in fact, today their team initiative is essentially defunct.

Common Barriers to Effective Communication

Understanding common barriers, such as gender and style differences, communication preferences, and tribal language, helps the
leader increase communication effectiveness.

Barrier One: Gender Differences

Anyone can see that there are differences between the genders. Not
so visually apparent, however, is one profound manner in which
men and women differ: communication. Differences in this area
have resulted from effects of the cultural environment and the way
people of each gender were socialized as children. Sometimes, however, we downplay these disparities in the workplace when attempting to emphasize similarities. Lack of appreciation for the
uniqueness of each gender only brings trouble for a leader attempting to communicate and establish relationships. In recent years a
plethora of popular books have discussed these differences. Any
leader interested in improving his or her communication skills
should read several of these books. This section identifies only a few
examples of gender-based differences and briefly examines leadership ramifications. Readers should consider none of the following
observations as absolutes for either gender but allow them to stimulate awareness and thinking about these differences.

Giving an Answer Versus Talking It Over

Young boys are socialized to give an immediate answer or solution to
a problem. Young girls talk things over to solve their problems. It does
not mean that the young girl wants an answer to the problem, just as
it does not mean that talking the issue over once is enough. Called
problem talk, these issues become great conversation for two women.
But when a woman starts talking over an issue with a man, a common initial reaction is for him to give her an answer (Tannen, 1994).
    John Gray, who wrote *Men Are from Mars, Women Are from
Venus* (1992), substantiates this. He says that men retreat, withdraw,

and in a sense, "go to their cave" (p. 30) when they have a problem. A man likes to work things out for himself, whereas a woman
likes to talk things over. In the workplace these two different
approaches can strain a leader-follower relationship. One way to
avert this problem is to state clearly at the beginning of the conversation what is desired. A woman might say to a male listener: "I
don't need an answer, I just want to talk about this, and I need for
you to listen." A man might ask a woman: "Do you want a suggestion here, or do you just want me to listen?" On the reverse side, a
woman who understands these differences will not take offense if a
man does not want to discuss an issue in depth. And when a woman
steps in to help a man (which may be normal and expected
coworker or team behavior), he may be insulted and believe she
thinks he cannot handle the situation himself.

A recent leadership team meeting clearly demonstrated this.
The team was composed of six women and one man. One was an
executive, and the rest were first-line managers in the hospital. Jim
was the manager of a department that was undergoing an extensive
implementation of a new computer system. Jim's department was
large, with over 120 employees reporting directly to him. Needless
to say, there was a great deal of confusion and more work than any
one manager could possibly handle. To exacerbate the situation, Jim
was a new manager.

At a leadership team retreat, the discussion revolved around the
upcoming implementation in Jim's department. Team members
were rapidly identifying problems, talking through issues, and suggesting solutions—including ways that they could help Jim with his
workload. The team grew more enthusiastic as the conversation
continued, and Jim grew more and more reserved. The retreat facilitator finally remarked on his behavior and stopped the process.
When the facilitator asked Jim how he was feeling about the offers
of help from his female teammates, he replied, "It feels like they
don't trust me to do my job." The female members of the team were
aghast and hurried to assure him. Jim had misconstrued their typi-

cally female response to help. After discussing the two different gender approaches, they sat back and asked Jim what he would like from them.

Separation Versus Attachment

In her book *In a Different Voice* (1982), Carol Gilligan reports the results of a longitudinal study of boys and girls that revealed some fascinating gender differences. In a study over many years, researchers completed each observation at five-year intervals. Gilligan points out that most children are still raised in their early years by female caregivers. Little boys, when they reach the age at which they become aware that they are physically different from their caregiver, learn to separate. So over the years, they become skilled at separating. Little girls do not have to separate from their same-sex caregivers, so they instead become very good at sustaining relationships.

This plays out in the workplace in potentially significant ways. Women are more likely to work hard at nurturing a relationship and working out issues in it, whereas men may be more likely to terminate a relationship rather than try to work it out. Another effect this can have is that men may more easily separate work from their relationships: even after a bitter battle in the workplace, the men involved will still go out and play golf together. For women, a major disagreement in the workplace can destroy a relationship.

Direct Versus Indirect Communication

Men are more comfortable making requests, whereas women are more likely to use indirect methods of communication. Many little girls are socialized to get what they want and need by hinting, indirectly asking, or using innuendo. A recent comic strip showed a wife asking her husband: "Ted, do you want to take my car to work today?" Ted then turns to their daughter and says: "What she really means is—it's low on gas, would you fill it up for me?"

In the workplace a woman who says: "I think the report is still out there on the desk" may actually mean: "Please bring it in."

Women may inadvertently hide the real message in so many words that a male coworker never gets it. There is usually no problem if two people who are direct, or two who are indirect, get together. The problem arises when the two different types get together.

Body Language

Body language may be different in the genders as well. Men talk most comfortably shoulder to shoulder, whereas women like to talk face-to-face. Deborah Tannen (1994) concluded that men may find a woman's direct face-to-face interaction to be flirtatious or intimidating. Gray (1992) found that when a man nods his head during a conversation, he means he agrees, whereas a woman nodding means she's listening. There's quite a difference between the meanings of these two signals.

As stated earlier, these are not absolutes. Cultural differences also affect each of these categories. However, if a leader does not understand these distinctions, significant miscommunication can occur. Exemplary leaders are translators, and the more they are aware of nuances in communication, the greater their effectiveness.

Barrier Two: Communication Styles and Preferences

A common barrier to effective communication is a lack of understanding or appreciation for differing communication styles and preferences. The excellent communicator pays close attention to a listener's style and adapts his or her own style accordingly. Some listeners want specific details and endless facts to support an idea or solution. Others get impatient with what they perceive as overkill and just want to get to the bottom line. Some followers are chatty and long-winded; others are reticent and seem unwilling to share more than one sentence at a time—delivered with a lot of effort! Some listeners are severely affronted and take it personally if others in the dialogue question their opinion or challenge their arguments. Others shrug off contradictory ideas and go about promoting their own opinion regardless of anyone else's viewpoint. None of these approaches is inherently right or wrong; they are simply different. The more the leader understands both his or her own personal style and the follower's communication style, the better able he or she is to avert problems.

Another communication technique that can help a person read another with greater sensitivity is called neuro-linguistic programming. It is based on research findings that people can be visual, auditory, or kinesthetic. Application of these findings to communication issues is obvious: a visual person better receives a message that is encoded with visual terminology; an auditory person, auditory terminology; and a kinesthetic person, kinesthetic terminology.

The trick is to listen for clues as to which of these the individual prefers. "One of the ways you can know this is by listening to the kinds of process words (the predicates: verbs, adverbs, and adjectives) that the person uses to describe his/her experience" (Bandler and Grinder, 1979, p. 15). A visual person's conversations include comments such as "I see what you are saying"; "Draw me a picture or map so I can see it"; and "Do you see what I mean?" An auditory person makes comments such as "I hear you"; "That rings a bell"; and "Let me hear it from your lips." A kinesthetic individual may say "I really feel for them"; "I can handle that"; or "It feels right to me."

Sophisticated communicators pick up these clues and begin to mirror the three preferences by including appropriately similar references in their messages. Rapport is easier to establish if the two parties use a shared language. All three of these sensory sources may be used in a consequential communication. Transmitting both in writing (for the visual person) and orally (for the auditory person), the leader should also deliver important messages with feeling.

Barrier Three: Tribal Language

In her book *Tribal Warfare in Organizations* (1988), Peg Neuhauser presents the concept of tribes as a source of major conflict in many organizations. For a leader, this has special ramifications. "In today's hospitals with their many specialized groups, each with its own vocabulary, executives who engender willing cooperation and build cohesive groups may well be the most highly skilled at speaking many special languages and at translating ideas captured in specialized, sometimes esoteric vocabularies into a common language that all organizational constituents can understand" (Henry and LeClair, 1987, p. 21). The highly effective leader has to be fluent in a multitude of languages in order to communicate constructively with followers.

In today's health care organizations, some of the tribes include but are not limited to administration, nursing, radiology, pharmacy, business office, environmental services, physicians, and security. Not only does the language vary from tribe to tribe, but so do the primary and important values, rules of the game, training and background, and thinking patterns (Neuhauser, 1988). These differences lead to conflicts and a lack of connection if the leader does not understand and take them into account when communicating.

Examples are common. Members of the laboratory tribe value accuracy over speed, whereas members of the accounts receivable tribe value speedy turnaround for bill payment. Rules of the game pertain to how the tribal members get the job done. Caregiving tribe members may believe that honesty with patients and families is the only wise policy and criticize what they perceive as political doublespeak by physicians or administration. The rites of passage for each tribe are very different, as is the education or training required. These rites for obstetric nurses may include passing state boards, working nights, or their first unassisted birth.

Lack of consideration for tribal differences leads to problems. For example, security officers need to be customer oriented, while they also play a primary role in an organization's safety and security. Whereas a caregiver or a receptionist may see the security officer's role as making people feel comfortable and welcome in the environment, the more urgently needed role in a large urban medical center may be to provide an intimidating presence in the emergency room. One organization, attempting to create multiskilled employees, encountered numerous problems in cross training security officers to also be transporters and care providers in its emergency department for this reason.

Language is a primary way in which tribes differ and one of the first things to cause trouble. A code in the medical records department is very different from what is also called a code in the intensive care unit. Each tribe has a language specific to its own culture. In the management information systems (MIS) department, there are bytes, memory, and megahertz. Simply calling the help line in MIS gives one a clue as to how different the languages are. If a leader does not understand a tribe's language, it is easy to inadvertently halt communication. Neuhauser (1988) describes this as the fifteen-second phenomenon: a member of one tribe meeting a member of another tribe usually insults the other within fifteen seconds. The impact on communication is obvious: it shuts down. The internal message that the listening member of the other tribe plays is: "He or she just doesn't understand us"; or "He or she is different from us." Referring to people from finance as number crunchers or bean counters can be demeaning. Telling patient-care providers that something is not in the budget is like waving a red flag. In the same way that becoming fluent in a foreign language allows one to communicate in another culture, so does understanding the many languages of the different health care tribes.

Health care tribes are so complex that the task of communicating without insulting requires tremendous effort. An individual may be a member of multiple tribes. Take, for instance, a nurse. Although there is a general nursing language, it is complicated by the specialty in which an individual practices. Obstetric nurses have different lingo from surgical or intensive care nurses. Home health and long-term care nurses have their own jargon. It may even differ by shift! Educators, regardless of original discipline, have their own language. Although the differences can seem overwhelming, a good leader makes the effort to become aware of these differences and works to understand each tribe.

Conclusion

This chapter has addressed one of the most crucial issues for any leader: how to communicate effectively. Without this skill, the other leadership competencies are virtually inoperative; relationships are not healthy; it is impossible to gain commitment to a cause; processes cannot flow smoothly; and the leader is unable to develop and nurture others. To be an effective leader, one must understand the various facets of spoken, nonverbal, and written communication and the barriers that must be overcome. Every day brings a leader numerous opportunities to improve his or her communication skills, as well as new challenges in creating shared meaning with followers.

Conversation Points

1. What types of communication problems do you see in your organization? What kinds of problems have they created?

2. What is the communication philosophy in your workplace? Is communication frequent, open, and timely? If you are a manager, how could you increase your communication with employees? What are the common thoughts or reasons you have for not communicating more fully with employees?

3. How effective are your listening skills? How often do you have other people repeat the same message you have already heard? Are you ever accused of not listening? What do you think are the behaviors that led to this accusation?

4. How comfortable are you using questions in conversations with others? How do others react to your questioning technique? Do your questions facilitate the flow of information? Do people open up more, or do they become more reserved and quiet?

5. In what ways do you use nonverbal language to enhance, rather than detract, from your messages?

6. Develop a list of etiquette tips for the use of e-mail and cell phones (the easy way to start is to list your pet peeves). Do you violate any of these when using these forms of communication technology?

7. What is your level of skill with written communication? What are the kinds of problems you experience? How could you improve your written communication?

8. What differences do you see in different people's communication styles? Which of these differences are related to gender, personal style differences, or tribal language?

5

The Art of Effectively
Facilitating Processes

*Solutions . . . reside not in the executive suite but in
the collective intelligence of employees at all levels,
who need to use one another as resources, often across
boundaries, and learn their way to those solutions.*
R. A. Heifetz and D. L. Laurie,
"The Work of Leadership"

Exemplary leaders are skilled at guiding key processes in order to obtain synergistic, extraordinary outcomes. Process facilitation is a critical competency for a leader because of the increasing complexity of today's work and the accelerating competency of workers. The old command-and-control approach to leadership and management was effective in the past when workers did not have the scope, skills, or ability to make decisions other than basic ones directly influencing their work. Today's workforce is better educated, more sophisticated, and increasingly interested in being involved in planning and making decisions that directly or indirectly affect their work. Ramifications for the present-day leader are significant. Good leaders develop relationships, gather input, involve others, guide discussions, build commitment, empower others, and recognize when a decision needs to be a group effort and then gain consensus. In short, they are capable and skilled at facilitating a variety of processes.

Facilitating processes as a leader is not as easy as it might at first appear. In the past managers were often rewarded for a get-it-done mentality and approaches that were decisive and outcome oriented. How they achieved a result mattered less than the fact that they did so. In fact, individuals who focused on the process involved in achieving outcomes often reached those results more slowly and were thus judged less effective. The current business climate adds pressure to managing processes in that it reinforces the need for quick action, decisive leaders, and an outcome-oriented approach. Courage is a necessary asset in a leader who is pressured for a decision but believes better results are possible when the leader and followers make a collective and collaborative decision.

In the first edition of this book, this chapter was titled "The Art of Effectively Managing Processes." The term *managing* implies that one can control the process, which discounts what we know of systems theory. An organization, a department, a team, an individual are all open systems. An *open system* is a system that continually takes in information, transforms it, and changes as a result. An open system is in a constant state of emergence. As such, emergent systems are anything but controllable, and our future is not just unknown but incapable of being known (Stacey, 1992). To the degree that the environment is stable and there is certainty about a particular outcome, there is a sense of control. Leaders understand that although our systems are continually in an emergent state, and thus unpredictable, wisely facilitating the inherent process unfolding can increase the certainty of outcomes.

This chapter explores several key tenets underlying the leadership skill of facilitating processes. The first is to understand and respect the process involved. The second tenet refers to the role of leaders in persistently seeking to improve current situations by continually challenging the process. The final tenet establishes the leader's role in facilitation. To illustrate, the chapter examines several fundamental processes as they relate to current health care leadership practice. These include empowering others, resolving conflict, creating teams, and facilitating the processes of change and transition. Chapter Six also includes the key process of problem solving but will discuss it with other approaches for getting needed results.

Tenet One: Understand and Respect Process

This tenet is twofold: not only must leaders understand basic processes that are operative in particular situations, but they must also respect the processes, allowing them to unfold in their own natural time frames. Both elements of this tenet are important. First, it is necessary to recognize the process involved and demonstrate knowledge of it through the application of logical, methodical, or other appropriate steps. A major cause of an ineffective process is skipping or eliminating an important step, as this chapter will illustrate.

Leaders need not always apply the steps to these processes in exactly the manner they are outlined here. Through practice, trial and error, and continual evaluation of outcomes, a leader gains experience and may develop his or her own processes. However, most processes have a structure that, when consistently applied, will improve outcomes.

Process requires patience. The leader and followers may spend more time in preparatory groundwork, but when they make decisions or formulate solutions, those involved are thoroughly committed to carrying them out. With the command-and-control approach, after the leader makes a decision or determines a solution, he or she must spend time convincing others to comply—a never-ending cycle of explanations, persuasion, and monitoring of behavior.

Respecting the process means that the leader understands approximately how long a normal process should take and allows the necessary time for the process to unfold naturally. This requires a significant amount of judgment because a little nudge or push may sometimes be required to get things back on track. When people express an aversion to processes, it likely comes from having had the too-frequent experience of involvement in a previous process that seemed never ending. People inexperienced or unskilled in facilitating processes sometimes let them drag on and on, never bringing closure or producing needed results. Following a process for its own sake is mind deadening and demoralizing. The purpose of managing process is to make it meaningful; and to be considered meaningful, a process must result in effective and beneficial outcomes.

Respecting process is similar to understanding and respecting the principles involved in a situation. Best-selling author Stephen Covey, in *Principle-Centered Leadership* (1990), describes principles as abiding laws of nature that never change. To explain, Covey uses farming as an example. A farmer cannot take it easy in the spring and summer—procrastinating and not planting—and expect a bountiful harvest in the fall. The farmer must plant the seeds in the spring and cultivate and fertilize the fields during the summer to be rewarded with a crop in the fall. Unable to hasten the growth of the crop or to control all the external elements that affect the crop's bounty, the farmer respects and awaits the unfolding of the process. In the same way, a leader who understands and respects the natural flow of a particular process does only what he or she can to influence results but knows that he or she cannot accelerate the process unnaturally or control it completely.

Examples demonstrating a lack of respect for process are common in today's health care organizations. Unfortunately, the external climate creates a sense of urgency and need that can easily affect the leader's ability or desire to patiently let a process unfold. Take, for example, the formation of a healthy relationship between followers and leaders. Establishing and maturing this relationship is a developmental process. It cannot be rushed or developed suddenly when a crisis generates a need for it. Yet observe what happens in an organization in which employees threaten collective action through a union-organizing attempt. The organization hires consultants to coach managers about what they can and cannot say. Overnight, managers are available and visible to employees, listening to what employees are saying and asking for input. It is often a matter of too little, too late. Employees often receive managers' sudden flurry of relationship building with cynicism. Worse, the managers' behavior may reinforce the thought that threatening union organization causes management and administration to listen to employees! The parties are more likely to resolve issues to their mutual satisfaction if they have established healthy relationships built on mutual trust and respect over the years. Leaders have always been listening to employees, and employees and managers work together as full partners. When a volatile or critical situation develops, followers will extend trust to a leader who has built a trusting relationship over time.

Numerous examples exist in the area of empowerment. One midsize hospital brought in consultants and paid hundreds of thousands of dollars for a reengineering and restructuring project in the 1990s. The project was believed to be essential for the organization's survival. Employees were cross trained and placed in teams and expected to assume responsibilities not only for their own work but for that of management and supervisory positions that the organization had eliminated. All this might have been reasonable except that the organization had never invested in employee or management education and development. Neither employees nor managers were prepared in any way for the tremendous change this project represented. The organization needed these people to be empowered yet had never taken time nor allotted resources to develop them. Instead of empowering and strengthening the organization, the initiative failed miserably; the hospital went on the market and later closed. Earlier investment in its people's development could have been the turning point for this organization's survival.

Tenet Two: Continually Challenge the Process

Leaders do more than simply understand the operative process and allow it to unfold within its natural time frame. Leaders continually question the process, looking for opportunities to improve it and methods that increase its effectiveness. "Challenge is the opportunity for greatness. People do their best when there's the chance to change the ways things are. Maintaining the status quo breeds mediocrity. . . . [Leaders] motivate others to exceed their limits. They look for innovative ways to improve the organization" (Kouzes and Posner, 1987, p. 29).

Challenging the process requires continually evaluating the effectiveness of outcomes and identifying lessons learned from the manner in which the outcomes were obtained. What went well, and what actions created problems? Did the process flow smoothly or drag on too long? Did the leader intervene at appropriate times? Was enough time allotted? Did members of the group or team participate fully?

Questioning the status quo results in opportunities for improvement. Too many times we do things in particular ways in an organization simply because we have always done them a particular way. A leader challenges this thinking by questioning the traditions: Does it make sense to continue doing things the old way? Is there a better way? Leaders are always on the lookout for something that is not working well or something that can be improved. Kouzes and Posner (1987, p. 32) clearly describe this role: "The root origin of the word lead is a word meaning 'to go.' This root origin denotes travel from one place to another. Leaders can be said to be those who 'go first.' They are those who step out to show others the direction in which to head. They begin the quest for a new order. In this sense, leaders are pioneers. They are people who venture into unexplored territory. They guide us to new and often unfamiliar destinations. People who take the lead are the foot soldiers in the campaigns for change."

Another way a leader challenges a process is to encourage risk taking. They take risks themselves and grow from the lessons they learn and the accomplishments they achieve. Leaders also encourage risk taking when they talk about their own failures and mistakes and treat these as opportunities for learning. They support followers when they make errors and expect them to learn from their mistakes. The overall attitude in the organization is similar to the sentiment that silent-film actress Mary Pickford expressed: "If you have made mistakes . . . there is always another chance for you. . . . You may have a fresh start any moment you choose, for this thing we call 'failure' is not the falling down, but the staying down" (*Quotable Women*, 1989, p. 22).

A risk is simply the act of seeking to achieve a goal that exceeds the usual limits. Risk is inherent in any change initiative or innovation. Exemplary leaders and followers are familiar with risk taking because it is part of their very nature. Uncertainty and danger are a normal part of this process. Taking a risk is central to everything worthwhile in life. A person cannot grow without taking a chance. In every risk there is an unavoidable loss, something that one has to give up in order to move ahead. Not risking is the surest way of losing. If an individual or organization continually shuns new experiences or experiments because they are risky, the result is a person or organization that is comfortable with fewer and fewer experiences. Not taking risks is a sure way to become stagnant and ill prepared for the future.

Part of a leader's role is to understand and become comfortable with risk taking. Although careful planning reduces risk considerably, no one is ever completely prepared to take a big risk. But we gain nothing if we venture nothing, of course. One of the changes today's managers most need is "to cultivate the imagination and courage to innovate—that is, to question received wisdom and constantly look for a better way. Too many managers are still afraid of innovation" (Kanter, 1997, p. 7).

Unfortunately, this is true not only of managers and employee leaders but also of many systems. Difficulty letting go of the hospital mentality and traditional modes of service can lead to an aversion to risk sharing among physicians, community agencies, and hospitals. Board members may also be averse to taking risks. Alan Gauthier suggests that board members have traditionally focused on narrow financial concerns and must now refocus and reorient themselves toward expressing the voice of the community (Chawla and Renesch, 1995). Their role is changing, and speaking for the community may mean accepting higher levels of risk for the system.

Tenet Three: Facilitating Process

In addition to understanding and challenging the process involved, the leader has a role in actually intervening to facilitate the process flow. Facilitation skills such as managing and leading group process, addressing difficult or negative group behavior, getting participation from everyone involved, asking the right questions, and guiding a group to consensus are necessary. However, a leader might use additional techniques to facilitate process. Teaching others the logical steps of a process is one technique. Rather than assuming that followers or participants understand the process involved, the leader encourages followers to learn the sequential steps and know what the leader expects. This smooths the process because followers become knowledgeable enough to actively support the process and can work in partnership with the leader.

Another subtle but critical manner in which a leader facilitates process is by providing the time needed to fully engage the process. The leader must be patient and thus encourages patience in others. The leader does not look for results too early yet urges progress based on realistic time frames and gives feedback that is reassuring and reinforcing. If the leader is a manager, this support can be very concrete, such as allotting time for employees to work through a process while being clear about expected outcomes. In a laboratory department, for instance, an employee action committee was working with another department on solving a particular problem. The manager not only approved employee time away from the department but assisted in finding replacement help for committee participants.

Removing barriers in the department or organization is another way a leader facilitates effective processes. This may be as simple as providing any training that followers need. Being clear about parameters, expectations, and levels of authority also reduces barriers. The leader may need to communicate and pave the way with other leaders or managers in the organization. Again using the example of the laboratory department, when the employee action committee was initiated, the leader made certain that several members were skilled in using an established problem-solving model. At the first meeting the leader taught other members of the committee the same model. The group established expectations and levels of authority for carrying out their responsibilities at the second meeting. The lab manager also contacted several peripherally involved department managers and introduced committee members to them, asking the managers for their support and assistance should committee members call on them.

This chapter has already briefly discussed the final way to remove barriers, which is to reduce risks involved in the process, using trial periods and properly measuring results. Expecting and planning for mistakes and stops and starts provides an opportunity for damage control. Modeling accepting behavior when mistakes occur and helping sort out the reasons for the mistake and ways to correct it removes yet another barrier.

These three tenets, or principles, can be applied to all types of processes. The specific processes necessary for today's leader to master include empowering or transferring responsibility to others, resolving conflict, solving problems, making decisions, creating teams, and managing change and transition. All are key elements to increasing a leader's ability to influence others in a manner beneficial to the organization and people involved. This chapter and the next will examine each process in some detail and will illustrate it with current real-life examples to show its importance, as well as common pitfalls.

Empowering Others

One of the most important processes that any leader can undertake today is transferring responsibility to others, often known as empowering them. Unfortunately, empowerment is also one of the least understood of the key processes. *Empowerment* became a buzzword in the late 1980s and early 1990s, but many never went beyond giving lip service to the concept. Use of the term today often brings cynicism and horror stories that seem to substantiate the ineffectiveness of empowerment. However, for leaders who found ways to operationalize the implied promise of empowerment, results have been dramatic.

The definition of *empowerment* is "to be given the legal authority to." The word *power* means "the ability to act or to produce a result." These two definitions combined are "to be given the legal authority to act or produce a result." Gibson (1991, p. 351) defines empowerment as "a social process of recognizing, promoting, and enhancing people's abilities to meet their own needs, solve their own problems, and mobilize the necessary resources in order for them to feel in control of their lives." This is very similar to the definition of *leader* that this book provided in Chapter One.

Empowerment is both a process and an outcome. As a process, the sequential order of steps in empowerment ensure a greater likelihood of success. Empowerment is dynamic because it is transactional, meaning that it occurs as a result of interaction between two or more people and cannot, therefore, be completely predictable. Empowerment is a developmental process because it is directly influenced by the increasing ability of an individual to accept higher and higher levels of responsibility.

We cannot overstate the importance of empowering people in organizations. Empowered employees are fully engaged in their work, contributing at a much higher level than their counterparts who see their work as simply a job. With the constantly shifting business climate and increasingly challenging external conditions facing health care, every organization needs the ability to respond rapidly. Quick response is virtually impossible from a workforce that has to constantly be told what to do, that is basically uninformed and unused to making decisions, and that has never participated in collaborative planning. On the other hand, organizations that have dedicated resources to continually developing their people and that treat their employees as intelligent partners in the delivery of services are much more likely to have individuals who are able to respond quickly when external and internal conditions change. These employees are not dependent on the manager or leader for direction or decisions; they can function independently and interdependently when they need to.

Many organizations develop and empower not just frontline employees but also first-line managers. This creates a tremendous ripple effect in the organization. Rosabeth Moss Kanter, a professor at Harvard Business School, has been on the frontier of management and leadership for nearly twenty years. She points out the dangers of *not* empowering managers in the organization: "Managers with power accomplish more because they have greater access to information, resources, and support in the company. Being busy, they pass the information and resources to subordinates. Thus, powerful leaders are more likely to delegate responsibility and reward talent. Powerless managers who can't easily get access to resources and information are frustrated and weak. The result is often petty, dictatorial managers who wield the only power they can: oppression of subordinates. It is powerlessness, not power, that corrupts" (1997, p. 6).

Empowerment does not occur simply because a leader says, "You are now empowered; go perform!" There is no Harry Potter magic wand to wave or incantation to pronounce so that people suddenly begin behaving differently. "Empowerment takes planning, patience, trust, and time. It's not something you can do overnight. If you want it to work, you have to commit to it. You must be willing to invest in it, support it with systems, and approach it in a logical, determined way" (McCarthy, 1997, p. 7).

The Process

As a process, empowerment begins with an understanding of four interrelated concepts:

- Capability

- Responsibility

- Authority

- Accountability

The sequential application of these four concepts leads to empowerment. First, let's clarify the meaning of each of these terms.

Capability

Capability refers to the ability, knowledge, and willingness of an individual to carry out the task, assignment, or responsibility. Ability is not only personal competence comprising skill and experience but the availability of needed resources. An individual may be willing to accept a particular responsibility but simply not have the time, equipment, or resources necessary to do an adequate job. Or vice versa: the person may have ability, both personal competence and resources, but lack willingness. All must be present, or empowerment fails.

Responsibility

Responsibility is the clear allocation or assignment of a task or piece of work to be accomplished. Responsibility also implies that the individual accepts this allocation. The person to whom the leader has given the task or assignment must accept ownership before this responsibility can truly be transferred. For instance, a team accepts responsibility for carrying out its work, monitoring and controlling work flow, and making necessary decisions within its members' scope of responsibility and authority. They are responsible for maintaining an acceptable standard and for continually searching for ways to improve their processes and outcomes.

Authority

Authority is the right to act in an area for which one has accepted responsibility. In order to carry out a responsibility, an individual must have a commensurate level of authority. According to Miller and Manthey (1994), there are four commonly accepted levels of authority:

> *Level One.* This is the authority to collect data or gather information. The individual takes no action on the data or information, and the person assigning the responsibility and granting the authority remains the decision maker.
>
> *Level Two.* Once the individual collects the data or information, he or she also reviews it and makes a recommendation based on his or her assessment and previous experience. The person assigning the responsibility and granting the authority continues to make the decisions but considers the gatherer's recommendation in making the final decision.
>
> *Level Three.* The individual collects and reviews the information, makes a recommendation, and discusses it with the person assigning the responsibility. After their discussion and agreement, the individual proceeds to carry out the action.
>
> *Level Four.* The individual can initiate independent action; he or she has the right to gather information, determine what needs to be done, and take necessary action. The person accepting the assignment has the authority to act in the place of the delegating individual.

In addition to these levels of authority, the individual's responsibility or authority may be limited by constraints or parameters of a particular situation. For instance, the individual may have responsibility for making a purchasing decision with a level-four authority but must stay within the constraints of an established dollar amount. Or a person may have the responsibility to make a decision and determine necessary action but only after getting agreement from certain key stakeholders.

Accountability

Accountability is the retrospective review of decisions made or actions taken to determine if they were appropriate. Did the decisions or actions achieve the desired outcomes? If results were not satisfactory, what corrective action would remedy the situation? This attitude of continual review is characteristic of a lifelong learner, a learning team, or a learning organization.

Applying the Process

When a leader applies this empowerment process sequentially, it goes something like this: before expecting a follower to take on a responsibility, the leader assesses the individual's ability and willingness. Does the person have the knowledge to carry out this responsibility? Are necessary resources, such as information and time, available? Has training or education been provided? Once the leader determines that capability is present, he or she clearly defines and communicates the responsibility. Assumptions are not enough; the assignment must be clear to both the party accepting the responsibility and the other people whom this assignment may affect. The parties discuss the applicable parameters and reach agreement on the appropriate level of authority. Finally, they determine outcome measures to monitor success.

The significance of empowerment as a developmental process is now clear. As an individual becomes more capable and highly skilled, the leader can give him or her more responsibility. The leader gradually increases the level of authority following successful performance of a responsibility. The leader may expand parameters and constraints as his or her comfort with an individual's performance increases. It would be highly foolish, and even dangerous, to give a novice performer a level-four authority and no constraints the first time that he or she takes on a responsibility.

This process appears simple, yet it contains pitfalls and may result in missteps for any health care organization today. When people feel disempowered, leaders can use this process to assess the source of the problem and give guidance for correcting it. Here are some of the more common examples of pitfalls with each of these elements of empowerment.

Pitfalls: Capability

Job requirements change as a result of new needs in the organization, yet people stay in their positions even though they are no longer able to do the work required. This leads to an environment of entitlement rather than earned authority. Organizations can communicate new expectations in the workplace, provide education and training, and give employees time to adjust and meet new standards. However, at some point organizations can expect these individuals to develop the abilities required or face a change in roles.

Another problematic situation occurs when individuals accept responsibility for something they are not capable of doing. Perhaps they believe they have the skills, but in reality they do not. This creates frustration for both parties, the individual and the leader. It also results in lengthy and potentially costly delays in completing the task.

Some individuals are simply unwilling to accept more responsibility. This creates an admittedly difficult situation for a leader or manager. With reductions in staffing levels and downsizing of organizations, everybody simply has to pull his or her own weight. The organization needs the highest levels of performance from every individual, and others cannot simply absorb shortfalls from those

not contributing fully. Although you cannot force someone to accept responsibility, you can make acceptance of responsibility a job
requirement; an individual who does not accept responsibility may
lose the job.

Also, there may be insufficient resources for people to capably accept certain responsibilities. Time, equipment, money, education,
training, or coaching may not be available, although individuals may
be willing to accept additional responsibility. Organizations that
attempted to convert to team-based structures in the 1990s are a
good example. They accomplished redesign of work and determined
team structures. They assigned employees to teams and expected
them to carry out their work in a new way without preparation in
the form of education or training; furthermore, the employees reported to managers who were inexperienced at and incapable of
coaching a team. This created a no-win situation for all involved.

Pitfalls: Responsibility

The most common pitfall with responsibility is that leaders do not
clearly communicate it but instead assume that followers understand
it. For instance, a manager-leader makes the mistake of assuming
that the job description clearly and completely defines what the
organization expects the employee to do. Leaders do not always realize that the position holder will be held accountable for numerous
other responsibilities and that the leader must clearly articulate
them. For instance, the leader should tell employees: "You are responsible for two things as an employee. The first is to do the work
for which you were hired at an acceptable level of quality. The second is to form and maintain healthy working relationships with
your coworkers as well as with your customers." This means employees, not managers, are responsible for relationship issues in the
workplace. This ranges from resolving conflicts in a positive manner to having open, honest, and direct communication with coworkers. Yet how many organizations have clearly and directly given
employees this expectation?

Another problem with the element of responsibility occurs when responsibilities overlap significantly. In one organization the chief operating officer (COO) was a cautious individual with a bad habit of asking multiple managers to do the same tasks. A manager whom the COO asked to investigate and follow up on a problem would discover that the COO had asked others to assume the same responsibility. The managers found this duplication of efforts irritating and demoralizing. In some rare instances, having several people share a responsibility makes sense. But in order to avoid a disempowering and discouraging situation, the involved parties need to clearly discuss who is doing what. Few people appreciate wasting time.

In some instances, individuals have an exaggerated sense of responsibility and take ownership beyond what the leader intended. This can also lead to frustration and discouragement for all involved. One organization created a team of internal trainers to provide the education and training for a major organizational initiative in process improvement. In the beginning the team mistakenly believed that its role was to lead this initiative. Team members felt responsible for the effort's success or failure; managers in the organization did not help matters when they abdicated their responsibility for leading the process. Conflict and difficulties were significant until each set of parties clearly defined its responsibility.

Pitfalls: Authority

Problems occur most frequently with the concept of authority. This area also causes the most confusion for people. Many individuals believe that empowerment occurs only when they have level-four authority and that anything less than independent action is disempowering. Nothing could be further from the truth. The level of authority has to be high enough for the individual to carry out the responsibility, and when these two are commensurate, empowerment results. Even a CEO or system president does not have level-four authority for every aspect of his or her work. In any role, some responsibilities rightfully entail a lower level of authority.

A second source of confusion around authority comes from the mistaken but commonly held belief that lower levels of authority are not as important. People in today's organizations make many mistakes and poor decisions because of this misconception. Leaders ask individuals to give their opinion or to gather information, but because they are not making the final decision, they do a halfhearted job of collecting or giving the requested information. The poor quality of the input creates a disadvantage for the individual making a final decision. Each level of authority is critical, and individuals must take seriously the responsibilities that come with each level of authority.

Both performers and leaders may falsely assume levels of authority unless they specifically discuss and agree to them. Conflict occurs when disagreement becomes apparent. Quality or problem-solving teams often run into this situation. In one organization this occurred in the nursing department with a very visible employee team that had been asked to develop a clinical career ladder for the department. The team worked diligently for months and created an entire program based on extensive research from other hospitals.

When the team was on the verge of implementing the program, the corporate human resource department stopped the process because of compensation issues and a need for equity across the entire system. The program included neither home health and long-term care nor other professional departments. This team had unwittingly exceeded its level of authority; as a result, a significant amount of resentment and frustration developed between the hospital nursing department, corporate human resources, and the rest of the system.

Changing levels of authority in the middle of a project is sometimes necessary but should be avoided if at all possible. A manager-leader may give an individual or a group a responsibility, and the parties may have agreed on its level of authority, only to have the manager-leader recall or decrease the level of authority when the individual or group does not carry out the work in the way the manager-leader expected. There are, however, multiple ways of achieving necessary outcomes; and a confident leader recognizes the need to relinquish control and let followers find their own way. Snatching a project or assignment away midstream may put off the followers and leave them unwilling to accept further responsibility.

New authority-related problems are appearing today with the major structural changes in the workplace. In the past, managers clearly had a certain level of authority and their reporting relationships were delineated and unambiguous. For many people in today's health care system, this has changed completely. Take, for example, the role of the nurse executive who is responsible for the nursing function throughout the system. The responsibility has become increasingly difficult to carry out now that it is dispersed among a variety of leader-managers, some of whom have no professional nursing background and may report directly to a different executive. Communicating the essence of nursing issues and ensuring quality standards in the absence of line authority requires strong leadership skills.

A final problem related to authority is the reversal of authority. This occurs when a leader undermines the work of an individual or group or simply shows a lack of respect for the final decision. This happens most frequently when the leader has neglected to identify key parameters up front, so the individual or group made the decision with incomplete information. Less frequently, the leader may have had no intention of relinquishing control but wanted others to feel as if they had participated.

In the early days of the quality movement, employees frequently learned this lesson the hard way. One quality team worked for six months on a specific problem. Its recommendation cost $200,000 to implement and included the addition of four full-time-equivalent positions to the annual personnel budget. No one had thought to tell the team that any recommendation could not exceed the current budget. Unfortunately, the experience led team members to conclude that administration was not serious about involving employees in decision making and that quality was not a primary concern. Although leaders had selected the team members because of their interest and commitment, they became unwilling after this experience to participate in any further projects. Sadly, these budget constraints might have been more acceptable to the team if leaders had identified them in the beginning stages of work.

Sometimes group members attempt to undermine decisions. A medical clinical affairs committee discovered this in one organization. The director of medical affairs was given the authority to solve a problem within a certain dollar amount. Two weeks later he reported on his actions. Two physicians who had not been present at the previous meeting began questioning and second-guessing his decision. The chair of the committee firmly reminded them that the committee had given the individual the authority to solve the problem and that it would respect and support his decision.

Pitfalls: Accountability

Although problems with authority are the most common, issues of accountability are often the most serious. This element may well be the weakest link in the chain. If organizations do not hold people accountable for their behaviors and actions, whatever they may do through the first three steps can be quickly negated. One reason so many things go right in organizations today is that many employees and leaders feel a high level of personal accountability, continually reviewing their outcomes and learning from them. People who are continual learners demonstrate a high level of internal accountability. Nevertheless, there are many problems with external accountability, that is, the formal, traceable lines of accountability in the organization.

Most organizations have only limited systems of accountability. Ascertaining what went wrong and why can sometimes be very difficult. Increasing numbers of part-time staff and per diem or temporary employees have made determining who is responsible when a problem occurs rather complicated. Assignments of employees are often not consistent, and many handoffs from caregiver to caregiver and department to department increase the difficulty of tracking.

Another issue hampering accountability is the tendency of managers and leaders to protect employees. When an individual or team makes a mistake or poor decision, the real role of the leader is to coach and support them in their efforts to correct the situation. Too often the manager steps in and takes responsibility for correcting the problem. Take, for example, a situation in which a physician goes to the manager-leader with a complaint about an employee or a team. If the manager takes care of the problem, the employee or team has learned little except that it is not capable of resolving its customer service problems. On the other hand, if the manager-leader coaches the individual or team to work directly with the physician to resolve the issue, both the team and the physician benefit. The manager's behavior is sometimes motivated by his or her satisfaction in solving problems or in some cases by expectations within the hierarchy. Many established bureaucracies have only limited tolerance for these situations and simply want them resolved in the quickest fashion possible.

The final major pitfall for accountability is that the consequences of mistakes or poor judgment are too often punitive rather than corrective. Many organizations blame and accuse people when things go wrong. These negative, punitive responses are probably the fastest way to squelch any desire to accept responsibility. People are quick learners, and they also watch what happens to their colleagues and coworkers. Swift retribution designed at extinguishing poor performance actually extinguishes all performance. Few people are willing to take risks in a harsh and unforgiving environment.

Summary

This process for empowering others is key to good leadership. It offers an effective mechanism for delegating responsibility and developing people. Without leadership's astute application of these skills, people in the organization are less likely to contribute at their highest potential.

Conflict Resolution

Conflict in the workplace is on the rise as major change disrupts comfortable and known routines, accelerated expectations require greater job performance, and the workforce shrinks as a result of changing demographics and work redesign and downsizing. People going through change and transition experience a wide range of intense emotional reactions, heightening the potential for conflict.

Common Reactions to Conflict

Most people react to conflict negatively for a variety of reasons. These include early socialization patterns, when parents admonished children for being angry or fighting with siblings, or past negative experiences with conflict. Perhaps the individual remembers how it felt as a child to hear his or her parents argue and fight with each other. If the arguments and conflict ended in physical abuse or divorce, the message the child retained may be that conflict is bad. On the other hand, if a child never saw or heard his or her parents disagree or argue with each other, the child might believe that conflict is to be avoided at all costs. The child may never have seen parents take steps for healthy conflict resolution and conclude that conflict does not exist in healthy relationships. Another factor influencing an adult's reaction to conflict is the normal need to feel in control of situations. Intense conflict is frightening for many because it is unpredictable and hard to control.

To effectively assist in resolving conflict, leaders with insight into their own reaction to conflict are an asset. Each leader has unique conflict resolution skills that are more highly developed. For instance, one leader may be especially skilled at mediating, whereas another may be a skilled negotiations coach. One may stay calm under attack, whereas another needs time away to separate emotions from interventions. Knowing and tapping into our strengths increases our ability to assist others.

Understanding and accepting one's limitations are also vital. Very few people enjoy being involved in open conflict, but a strong leader recognizes that conflict is part of everyday life in any organization or workplace; every relationship has within it the elements of potential conflict. People often avoid conflicts because emotions run high; egos respond to attack; people feel hurt; and solutions seem elusive and difficult to reach.

The Positive Side of Conflict

When we consider conflict a normal part of the environment, it takes on a more positive aspect. Teams, for instance, go through a normal stage of development called storming in which the predominant characteristic is conflict. Members argue about everything, disagree with the team leader and each other, and resist even good ideas. Healthy teams learn how to resolve conflict from these experiences as they work out these issues together. The team becomes stronger by confronting and addressing differences and conflicts rather than avoiding or ignoring them. What is true for teams is also true for individuals. Too many people believe that avoidance is the best approach for dealing with conflict, but all it does is delay the inevitable—the need to deal with the conflict.

Conflict can serve as a positive, driving force for change and improvement. It often exposes true feelings, which leads to a better frame of mind and increases the likelihood that resolution will occur. When one party shares true feelings, it allows others to understand how strongly that individual feels. Open conflict can save time in an organization because excessive politeness and courtesy may mean that the parties accomplish nothing. Conflict over procedures, policies, or systems in place forces examination of the status quo. Conflict helps us identify our boundaries more clearly. We usually experience conflict when someone has impinged on something important to us. Maybe something needs to change in order to prevent a serious problem later. An honest dispute often engenders a greater mutual respect among individuals and a clearer understanding of the positions of both sides. Seeing others disagree and work out conflicts encourages the more timid to express their opinions, which they might otherwise have never shared.

The benefits of open conflict were demonstrated clearly by a clinical information systems team in a midsize hospital in the South. For the first six months, the team members worked beautifully together, becoming a strong team and establishing their purpose and working approaches. At this point, however, a major conflict about working approaches erupted during a team meeting in which the external leader-manager was not present. The team had agreed on a specific procedure for documenting help calls received from customers that would allow the team to measure outcomes and evaluate their service. One team member, the laboratory's computer systems person, continued to document her help calls in the manner she had been accustomed to prior to the team's formation, thus creating problems for the team in tracking their outcomes.

When the rest of the team discovered this, open conflict exploded between this individual and other members; the team spent the entire meeting trying to work through this issue. Weeks later they still expressed negative feelings about the conflict and believed that they should have handled the situation better. In exploring these feelings, the leader asked the team to identify what they had learned from the situation. They came up with thirteen specific things that were positive about either how they had handled the conflict or what they had learned from the experience. This discussion immediately shifted their perception from "conflict is bad" to "conflict can help us grow."

The Leadership Role

In organizations that empower employees, those employees assume responsibility for having healthy relationships with others in the workplace, which means being responsible for effective resolution of conflicts. In organizations with teams, team members are responsible for resolving conflicts that occur. In both instances, however, employees need a leader to coach them as they learn these skills and at times to serve as mediator. The leader's role is to develop others in their conflict resolution skills and intervene only as necessary. The leader carefully assesses the situation and does not hesitate to intervene when the situation requires the use of the manager's legitimate authority, such as in cases of bullying. Employees can be taught skills to deal with bullying behavior; however, extreme examples may require intervention from management and even human resources staff. Leaders use a variety of approaches for conflict resolution and should avoid those that are only partially effective.

Ineffective Methods of Conflict Resolution

Some methods of conflict resolution are ineffective. These strategies may seem effective over the short term, but because the solution is not mutually beneficial to the involved parties, not all are committed to supporting the solution. Strategies that appear to solve the conflict but instead produce frustration, distrust, and a feeling of being treated unfairly include

- Competition
- Coercion
- Intimidation and dominance
- Persuasion
- Procrastination and avoidance
- Coalition building
- Accommodation

Competition

Competing is an ineffective strategy for resolving conflict because it encourages a scarcity mind-set in which there is never enough (time, resources, financial support) to go around. It creates a win-lose rather than a win-win situation. The parties do not even consider sharing for mutual benefit when individuals or teams are pitted against each other; for one to win, the other must lose.

Coercion

Either overt or covert coercion seems to settle the matter quickly but actually results in resentment. Leaders must be careful when serving as mediators not to use coercion. Because the leader-manager has legitimate authority, the leader's expression of an opinion can feel like coercion to others. This legitimate authority can give unfair weight to the manager's opinion. Coercion can also occur among peers. One individual may feel coerced into accepting a disagreeable point of view in the interest of preserving harmony within the group.

Intimidation and Dominance

Similar to coercion, intimidation and dominance are pressure tactics based on power relationships. In the short term, they may seem to be effective, but many people find them distasteful. Intimidation and dominance can destroy trust in a relationship because of use of unfair advantage.

Persuasion

Persuasion is a strategy that articulate, charismatic people commonly use. The problem with persuasion is that the persuader ends up psychologically superior to the persuaded individual. When an individual uses persuasion, keeping people focused on the solution becomes more and more difficult over time. Greater doses of persuasion are needed as people begin thinking for themselves and questioning the solution they were persuaded to accept.

Procrastination and Avoidance

Putting off any real resolution of the disagreement or conflict is the basis of this strategy. It usually causes the conflict to feed on itself and become worse with time. People often use a short delay in dealing with the conflict to see whether it will work itself out. Although this is appropriate and effective in some instances, leaders should use delays in addressing conflict judiciously and not allow them to interfere with effective resolution of the conflict.

Coalition Building

Alliances, in the positive sense, are often needed to get something accomplished. As a means of resolving conflict, however, building coalitions can be negative because it forces people to choose sides. This increases the likelihood of head-to-head battles. Unfortunately, this is one of the more common approaches to resolving conflict in health care today. Employees who feel unable to obtain what they need through their own efforts talk to physicians in an attempt to engage them in the cause. Department managers in conflict with one another often talk to other managers in an attempt to build support for their positions. Some actually view this as an effective executive strategy: getting all their ducks in a row before a key meeting. Purposely talking with others to bring them to a certain point of view is building a coalition, which may work well when the group is planning or making a decision. But it is ineffective over the long haul in resolving active conflict.

Accommodation

Accommodation is a strategy that is helpful at times but is easy to overuse. It means that one party is giving up its rights or desires and allowing the other's rights or desires to take precedence. In some instances, this may be appropriate in order to benefit the whole. One problem with accommodation is that the same individual or group tends to allow this and eventually grows to resent the situation. Accommodation can result in perceptions of uneven status and foster long-term resentments. Individuals who usually seek harmony may begin to feel that others are taking advantage of them.

Effective Methods of Conflict Resolution

Although in the real world a perfect solution to conflict simply does not exist, parties in conflict can attempt several potentially effective strategies. These enable the parties to deal with the conflict in an open, positive manner while limiting the conflict's negative impact. Effective methods of resolution include the following:

- Appeal

- Mediation

- Superordinate goals

- Peaceful coexistence

- Negotiation

Appeal

This strategy allows any party to take a decision to a higher level or to someone who is not emotionally or directly involved with the situation. Appeal is powerful because when both parties in a conflict realize that they can appeal a decision, it inspires them to seek resolution more honestly. The grievance procedure that exists in most organizations is a good example of an appeal process. However, a team or individuals can use it more informally by simply agreeing to take the decision to an uninvolved third party for a decision. When using the appeal, both parties must agree to support the third party's decision.

Mediation

Although similar to appeal because it involves a third party, mediation is different. It requires the involvement of a knowledgeable and trusted third party to act as an intermediary for all involved in the conflict. The mediator's objective viewpoint can often diffuse emotions and serve as a catalyst to reach a mutually agreeable solution. When the leader serves as a coach or facilitator for conflicting parties in a conflict, this is an example of mediation. In some instances, each party has its own coach.

Superordinate Goals

Finding a goal that transcends the special interests of both parties is an excellent strategy for resolving conflict. This is a superordinate goal, which leaders use frequently, perhaps without even realizing it. Asking people to forgo minor differences and stay focused on the overriding purpose and goal is an example of this approach. The urgent deadlines and immense challenges facing a work group often pull them together and facilitate the speedy resolution of conflicts that arise.

Peaceful Coexistence

This strategy is useful in selected situations when the parties in conflict can stay on their side of the fence without negative impact. If two employees, for instance, find each other abrasive, they can still agree to work together peacefully if there is some separation, such as working on different shifts or in different departments or not having a significant amount of interdependent work to do. The leader gets the involved parties to agree to the old adage of "I don't have to like you to work well with you." This approach works only if the parties establish clear expectations and agree to work within them. These attitudes must not affect the work group's level of activity.

Negotiation

Probably the most effective strategy for resolving conflict is negotiation. This strategy is based on a win-win problem-solving approach, in which no one involved has to give up anything that is essential to him or her. Negotiation is a process of mutual agreement. It is approached from a win-win stance and takes place with a spirit of cooperation rather than conflict. Negotiation is the most powerful strategy for conflict resolution simply because in any work situation, the parties involved are likely to interact with each other over the long term. If they find win-win solutions, each party will be committed to supporting these decisions. If one of the ineffective strategies is used, such as coercion, a subsequent conflict among the same people will be much more difficult to resolve. The party who lost in the first round is likely to be waiting for the next opportunity to get even.

Nierenberg and Ross (1985) outline a specific process for negotiating that they refer to as a negotiation map. On this map the steps for negotiating a conflict are the following:

1. Define the issue.
2. Clarify objectives.
3. Gather all relevant information.
4. Identify alternatives.
5. Select strategies.

Step One: Define the Issue. The need to define the real issues in a negotiation may seem self-evident, but a good negotiator makes no assumptions. For example, when a team and manager are experiencing conflict about a decision that the manager has made, the real issue may not be the outcome or decision but the fact that the manager made the decision rather than allowing the team to do so within clearly identified parameters. These are two very different issues; the real issue may be the team's decision-making authority.

The first step is to determine that both sides of the dispute share an understanding of the issue. This requires honesty and the ability and willingness to disclose hidden agendas. Both parties must trust each other enough to share information openly, without fearing that the other party will use the information in an adversarial manner. Hidden agendas and personal issues can destroy individuals' ability to effectively negotiate.

One newly formed senior leadership team was in the process of negotiating its members' assignments when a hidden agenda blocked their progress. Five new executives had been appointed but were not yet assigned to specific care centers. In a meeting to determine division of responsibility, one of the new team members, Lynette, was operating with a hidden agenda: she did not want to be assigned to a particular care center. Throughout the discussion every comment and suggestion Lynette made was based on her avoiding taking an assignment to that particular care center rather than focusing on what was best for the organization. The meeting ended in a stalemate with Lynette in tears. Her teammates were flabbergasted because the decision was not emotional in nature to them and they were not sure what was happening. The team decided to think about the possibilities over the weekend and return on Monday to further discuss the issue prior to making a decision.

When the facilitator talked with Lynette and discovered the important personal agenda she was keeping hidden, she advised Lynette to be open with her teammates and share her strong feelings. When she did so, the team was able to rapidly reach a decision that was good not only for the organization but for each team member.

Step Two: Clarify Objectives. In this second step on the map, each party determines what it desires. This sounds somewhat simplistic, but people often limit themselves by limiting their objectives. Thinking broadly about objectives may extend the possibilities available to consider in negotiation. Each side may have a range of objectives that would be satisfactory.

An example of this arose during the annual performance appraisal of an excellent department secretary in a home health agency. Renee was a superbly skilled secretary but functioned more as a direct assistant to the administrator of a special program. During her annual review, she requested a promotion to an executive assistant position. The manager knew this was impossible in the current setting because the agency could have only one executive assistant position. In talking with Renee, the manager asked why she was interested in the promotion. Was the title important, the increase in pay, the type of work included in the job? Renee's response was interesting: she had noticed that the executive assistant was the only secretarial or clerical person who attended workshops and seminars at the company's expense. Renee valued continuing education and wanted the same opportunity. Fortunately, this was something that the manager could provide, so once they had identified this objective, they easily achieved a win-win solution.

Step Three: Gather All Relevant Information. This next step includes gathering any relevant facts, identifying operative assumptions, and determining needs of the involved parties. Facts are important because they determine how negotiable certain positions are. The more facts the parties share, often the more successful the negotiation. Checking out the assumptions of all parties is absolutely critical because people often make decisions based more on assumptions than on facts. Both before and during an active negotiation, both parties sharing openly what they need increases the likelihood of a successful win-win negotiation. Parties should not confuse priority needs with peripheral needs. For negotiation to have lasting results, both parties must have their priority needs satisfied so that each has a stake in the continued success of the solution.

When a physician asked a laboratory manager to have lab results available for early morning rounds, she discovered that to draw the lab specimens early enough, patients would have to be awakened before 4 A.M.! Most patients would be highly dissatisfied by this early awakening. Furthermore, although the physician had made it sound like one that many physicians wanted, investigation revealed that only one or two other physicians had been involved in the request. Another false assumption was the physicians' belief that this request would have no effect on the budget. Also, in terms of needs, it initially appeared to require a major shift in the laboratory employee's schedule. But the manager checked the facts and discovered that the physicians really needed this only on Sundays, when the physicians involved wanted to attend early church services and therefore to make rounds earlier than usual.

Step Four: Identify Alternatives. In this step, the parties consider all possible alternatives. As when identifying objectives, widening the range of possibilities makes finding a mutually acceptable solution more likely. After brainstorming to uncover all options from both parties, it is appropriate to begin to whittle them down to acceptable alternatives.

In the previous example of the lab manager and the physicians requesting earlier lab reports, the parties considered numerous ideas. Was there a technological fix? Was the lab already considering newer, faster equipment? Could floor or lab employees change schedules easily enough? Was no change actually best for all involved? Could lab services be decentralized or redeployed to smaller, more local labs nearer the patient units?

From the list of possible alternatives, generate at least two, and preferably three, reasonable alternatives. Locking on to only one acceptable alternative can be a trap in negotiation because it results in an ultimatum. Multiple alternatives allow for true choice.

Step Five: Select Strategies. Once you have identified acceptable alternatives, determine the action to take. Strategies are the actions to be taken both during and after the negotiation and include the type of climate to set for an effective negotiation. Climate should be fluid and dynamic in every negotiation. Nierenberg and Ross (1985) believe that the party controlling the climate has more influence over the negotiation and that the other party generally accepts positive climates and resists negative climates.

The lab manager in the previous example, for instance, thought through the information she had and how to present it to the physicians. Part of her strategy might have been to discuss their needs more fully and to share the assumptions she discovered. Sharing the facts she had collected might have helped appeal to the physicians' logic. She probably also considered strategies for establishing a positive climate. Would the discussion take place in her office, the physician's office, the hospital dining room?

This negotiation map works best when it is treated as a dynamic process. To prepare for a negotiation, each individual works through the map first from his or her own perspective and then from the other party's perspective. The most effective negotiators are those who are clear about their own positions, not overly accommodating, yet flexible when the other party has a valid point. Parties most easily assume this role when they have fully considered each step of the negotiation process. Clear expectations between the parties for obtaining a win-win situation can result in effective negotiation. In the Grand Forks, North Dakota, system integration case example in Chapter Three, the law firms for the parties involved were both told they must find a win-win solution. This powerful message clearly avoided the development of adversarial posturing and positioning.

Pitfalls of Conflict Resolution

The most common pitfall related to conflict resolution is a tendency to avoid dealing with conflict. Although few people approach a conflict situation with enthusiasm, some individuals absolutely abhor conflict of any kind and thus greatly reduce their effectiveness because they simply won't deal with it or they become immobilized in the face of conflict. Modeling this behavior as a leader sends the wrong message to followers, who will think: *If the leader cannot effectively deal with conflict, why should we bother?*

The experience of one health care entrepreneur is a good example of this pitfall. A visionary head of his own company, Bob had attained great success. However, his Achilles' heel was an inability to deal with conflict. In his organization he had retained several costly employees who consistently underperformed, yet he dreaded confronting them over their lack of performance. Not only did they contribute significantly to a high overhead, but the company lost several excellent performers who were not willing to continue to work hard to cover the nonperformers' salaries.

Bob worked diligently to expand the company's services, and one strategy involved partnering with other companies. These relationships began with great enthusiasm and high hopes, but at the first sign of any conflict (and what relationship is without it?), Bob would withdraw his support and sever the relationship. Needless to say, the company's reputation began to deteriorate. The source of all of these problems was Bob's intense discomfort with conflict and the resultant inability to deal with it effectively.

A second common pitfall exists when a leader is so emotionally attached to an outcome that objectively identifying possible alternatives becomes difficult or impossible. Too often these situations reach an impasse, at which point one party delivers an ultimatum. This is rarely, if ever, a healthy way to resolve conflict. A midsize hospital in the Southwest averted such an impasse. Liz, the vice president of patient services, had the explicit trust of John, the CEO to whom she had reported for years. John supported her decisions and valued her judgment. On this occasion a recruiting process for a new director of perioperative services was under way. Liz saw no viable internal candidates, and recruiting efforts had brought forth only two external possibilities. Suddenly, a couple of the anesthesiologists decided they would recommend one of the operating room staff nurses for promotion. The suggestion fell on deaf ears: Liz felt the individual was not qualified for this promotion for a number of valid reasons. When the physicians were unable to achieve their goal through Liz, they descended on John's office. Although John sent the physicians back to Liz, he also talked to Liz directly about the recommendation and came very close to telling her to hire the internal candidate. Although Liz did not tell him directly at this point, her immediate response was concern that if John told her she must hire this individual, Liz felt she would have to resign. She did not believe she could continue in her position if John interfered in such a way with her authority.

After discussing the situation with an objective and trusted colleague, Liz identified several alternatives that helped prevent the situation from escalating into an out-and-out conflict. Liz set up an interview process that included employees, other managers, surgeons, and anesthesiologists. They identified selection criteria ahead of time, and interviewers evaluated each candidate for the position against these measures. As a result, the anesthesiologists realized for themselves the limitations of the internal candidate they were promoting.

The final major pitfall with significant consequences is seeing conflict only in a negative light. This creates an organizational culture in which people do not express disagreements openly because of fear that they may damage a relationship; staff repress conflicts; and people do not express their honest reactions to ideas or events because of possible repercussions. When this is the organizational culture, managers and leaders have little experience using the effective methods of conflict resolution because they view conflict as something to avoid at all costs.

This described the organizational culture in one eastern seaboard medical center that was part of a large system. One of the system's four hospitals underwent a major work-redesign initiative. Planning took two years, with employees and key stakeholders heavily involved. Implementation of the new design began on the first two patient-care units and, as is normal during major change, multiple conflicts arose. Implementation did not proceed as smoothly as anticipated, and physician and patient complaints increased. Some saw the conflicts as a sign that the change was not working, and the chief operating officer pulled the plug on the entire project! Years of work and hundreds of thousands of dollars were lost because the conflict was interpreted as failure rather than a normal step along the process. The impact on leadership credibility in the organization was also quite significant.

Creating Teams

Creating and developing high-performance teams is another key process that today's leaders must master in order to be effective. "Teams make sense in today's world for many reasons: the increasing complexity of our work; the changing values of the workforce; the increasing need for immediate organizational response to difficult external marketplace changes and internal challenges; and our desire to create a healthy, satisfying workplace for employees" (Manion, 1997, p. 31). Exemplary leaders understand the concept of the team and determine when a team can do a better job than an individual. Even more important, effective leaders have the skills to facilitate a team's development.

Team and *teamwork* are terms that people often confuse and use as synonyms, but they are two different concepts. The word *team* is overused today, loosely applied to exhort others to perform in a particular manner, usually through teamwork. *Teamwork* is a way of working together, and it may mean different things to different people. For most, it implies cooperation, open communication, and pitching in to help each other out. A *team*, in contrast, is a structural unit, a group of people designed and drawn together to complete certain prescribed work. How team members carry out the work can be described as teamwork. As adapted from Katzenbach and Smith's definition in *The Wisdom of Teams* (1993), a team is "a small number of consistent people with a relevant, shared purpose, common performance goals, complementary and overlapping skills, and a common approach to its collective work. Team members hold themselves mutually accountable for the team's results and outcomes" (Manion, 1997, p. 31).

Organizations today have several types of teams:

- Primary work teams
- Ad hoc teams
- Leadership teams

Primary work teams are permanent structures organized around a department's primary work. In a business office, the teams may be organized around business functions, such as credit verification, billings, and collections. Teams in a patient-care department are organized around patient care. For example, teams in a laboratory are often designed around specialized functions, such as microbiology, hematology, and chemistry. The emergency department may have a trauma team or urgent-care team. *Ad hoc teams* are temporary teams created to perform a particular piece of work; after the work is completed, the team is dissolved. Quality or continuous process improvement and project teams are good examples of ad hoc teams, which can last for years and yet not be considered part of an organization's permanent structure. *Leadership teams* are formed to provide collective leadership for a project or initiative, department, service, or organization.

Leaders today may need to create a team for a specific purpose (such as sharing the leadership function for the department), may actually redesign their department into teams, or may have shared responsibility for guiding or participating in the conversion of the bureaucracy to a team-based structure. Other sources discuss the implementation of teams in health care extensively (Manion, Lorimer, and Leander, 1996; Manion, 1997; Lorimer and Manion, 1996; Leander, Shortridge, and Watson, 1996; Manion and Watson, 1995). Exemplary leaders who understand the concepts and language of systems thinking often form diverse teams that use systems thinking to focus on critical issues. These teams outperform individuals because systems issues require multiple approaches, a variety of experiences, and diverse thinking patterns.

Regardless of the type of team, there are concrete steps to use in creating an effective team.

Step One: Define the Work

Prior to selecting team members, the leader must define the work he or she expects of the team. The individual initiating a team delineates what the team is expected to do by considering certain questions: What is the primary work this team is to accomplish? Is this a problem-solving team focusing on a specific issue or a project team formed to design and implement a new service or system? Is the team's work to provide collective leadership for the department or for the organization? What will be required of this team? Is systems thinking required to challenge mental models and initiate breakthrough thinking? What are the general goals and objectives of this group? This step can be difficult, but it forces the leader to be very clear about his or her reasons for initiating a team.

Step Two: Select Members

Based on the work the team is to do, potential members are identified. Members are selected based on their potential contribution to the team's work. The team member may represent a particular part of the system or have certain skills that the team needs. In some cases, it is impossible to obtain all the skills the team needs, and members may be selected for their skills potential; then development of those skills is paramount. Perhaps no one in the organization has exactly the skills needed, but the team can develop those skills through its work.

The most effective teams are those with a small number of consistent team members. Teams of more than twelve members simply run into more logistic problems than do smaller teams. In larger groups, members too easily disengage and remain anonymous. Finding a common time to meet is more problematic with larger groups. Consistency of membership is critical. Frequent changes in team membership directly affect the group's synergy and the quality of work team members complete. When team members leave and are replaced, the team usually regresses in its effectiveness until the new member is brought up to speed and is fully assimilated into the group. Consistency of membership also refers to consistent attendance at team meetings. Frequent absenteeism directly affects the team's ability to produce high-quality outcomes.

Step Three: Define the Team Purpose

Once the team comes together for the first time, the initial work of the team is to define its purpose. Although the leader may have given the group some preliminary direction (based on his or her thoughts from step 1), it is critical that the team develops its own mission or purpose statement. This describes what the team does and for whom. It clarifies the reason for the team's existence. Teams that are handed a completed purpose statement, or are simply told by the leader why they exist, never develop the same level of ownership as those teams that actually do this work. If the team is given a mission statement describing its work, one way to ensure relevancy and identification with this purpose is to have the team modify it to fit its beliefs. Even small modifications increase team members' feeling of ownership. Team members simply do not engage with the work if they do not find the team's purpose relevant.

It is important for the leader to stay involved with the team during development of this mission statement in order to prevent the team from heading in the wrong direction. The team's purpose must also be congruent with the organization's or department's purpose. If the two are incongruent, the team is headed for trouble. An actively participating leader does not mandate the team's purpose but is involved in guiding and setting the general direction.

Step Four: Establish Common Working Approaches

Once the team is clear about its mission and reason for existence, the next step is to determine and agree on the approaches it plans to use in doing its work. "A common approach means that team members discuss, delineate, and agree on ways they are going to work together to accomplish their purpose. Common refers to the collective effort that is required, not an approach that is ordinary or average. There is nothing common nor ordinary about a highly effective team" (Manion, Lorimer, and Leander, 1996, p. 64).

Some examples of early decisions to make about working approaches include the following:

Logistics of team meetings. How often will the team meet? When will it meet? Where? Will an agenda be circulated? How is the agenda developed? Who facilitates the meeting? Will minutes be needed? If so, who will take them?

Methods for communicating. This includes both formal and informal methods of communicating. Is there a need for frequent team huddles? Are team members readily accessible to each other? Do they need to be? How will they communicate between meetings? Is everyone on e-mail?

Problem-solving approaches. How will the team tackle problems? Is there a specific quality improvement process the team must follow?

Decision making. What types of decisions will the team make? What are the boundaries in regard to the team's work? Which will be individual decisions, and which should the entire team make? Will the team make decisions by majority vote or by consensus? When will a subset of the team be authorized to make decisions instead?

Doing the work. Are there certain processes and approaches the team agrees to do a certain way? Does there need to be consistency in practices? (In the conflict resolution section earlier in this chapter, the clinical information team that agreed on how to record the help calls members received is an example.)

The team also needs to discuss members' roles and responsibilities. Do team members need to fill specific roles to ensure that work is completed? Examples of these include meeting coordinator or facilitator and process person. Some teams identify a celebrations role to ensure that the team recognizes and cheers key events and accomplishments. If there are any needed roles, the team must define specific responsibilities of each role clearly. Some teams identify the role of challenger. The challenger is "the team member who openly questions the goals, methods, and the ethics of the team, who is willing to disagree with the team leader, and who encourages the team to take well-considered risks" (Parker, 1997, p. 8). This role is critical for most teams because the challenger is honest in reporting team progress and identifying problems. This individual, however, backs off and actively supports consensus within the team if the team does not accept his or her views. In other words, this person is not always in an adversarial role. Another common role is the team recorder, who generates the minutes of meetings and circulates them; this is often a rotating responsibility.

The final components of establishing common working approaches are the discussion of and agreement on what team members expect of one another. Identifying and articulating behavioral expectations are key steps early in team formation for several reasons. These expectations lay the foundation for development of trust within the team. In addition, being clear about the expectations one holds of others is instrumental in preventing unnecessary conflicts. Too often people do not meet others' expectations because they did not know the expectations even existed. The group discusses what members expect or need from one another in order to do a good job. This often includes expectations for appropriate meeting participation, communication techniques, and acceptable team behavior. The following example from a real team demonstrates expectations related to these areas:

> We expect team members to
> - Be on time and prepared for meetings and to fully participate as evidenced by an attentive attitude, asking clarifying questions, and remaining open-minded about the contributions of other team members
>
> - Communicate openly, honestly, and directly with each other, especially if we fail to meet each other's expectations

- Work toward the goals of the team and support the success of the team first and individual work second

- Stay focused on our goals and complete tasks and projects within agreed-upon time frames (communicating any unavoidable delays to other team members as soon as possible)

Clear expectations help formalize the team's norms, one of the first steps in building and creating the team's emotional intelligence (Cherniss and Goleman, 2001). Being willing to address another team member's failure to live up to established norms and expectations is a crucial sign of the team's emotional intelligence. Fear of conflict and confrontation is a common dysfunction of ineffective teams. Seen as accountability, team members' willingness to call their peers on performance or behaviors that might hurt the team and its performance is essential for effective functioning (Lencioni, 2002).

Step Five: Specify Performance Goals

Closely related to the team mission are the team's performance goals. Larson and LaFasto (1989) examined high-performing teams and found, without exception, that these teams had clearly identified performance objectives and goals. These can also serve as a measurement of the team's outcomes, giving a team the ability to hold itself accountable.

Team goals are distinguished from system, organizational, or department goals. "Teams take broad objectives or directives from the organization's management and shape them into specific, measurable goals for the team. Specific goals are stated in concrete terms so that it is unequivocally possible to tell whether or not they have been met" (Manion, Lorimer, and Leander, 1996, p. 63). The most powerful goals provide for small wins along the way, and these intermediate victories serve to motivate and reinforce the team's direction along its chosen path.

Motivating goals are often those with stretch, forcing the team to extend itself and reach beyond what it had previously dreamed of. These ambitious goals produce momentum, growth, and commitment within the team. "Teams that face a significant challenge, or that develop their own ambitious goals, have a greater sense of urgency that forces them to focus their efforts in a unified direction. . . . The true strength of a team is realized when it faces and overcomes seemingly unbreachable obstacles to attain a worthy goal" (Manion, Lorimer, and Leander, 1996, p. 63).

Step Six: Hold the Team Accountable

A final and essential step is to hold the team accountable for its outcomes. This is a constant process of reviewing outcomes and determining whether the team has met established standards and obtained expected outcomes. If the team has not obtained desired outcomes, it evaluates its process and its work to determine what went wrong and then takes corrective action.

"Mutual accountability differentiates a real team from a working group. In both teams and working groups, individuals hold themselves accountable for the outcomes of their assignments. A team, however, takes the next step—members hold themselves mutually accountable for the team's outcomes or results. They continuously measure themselves against their established goals and objectives" (Manion, Lorimer, and Leander, 1996, p. 77). The team reviews its decisions for effectiveness and its processes for beneficial outcomes. All team members are equally accountable for the team's outcomes.

Leadership Teams

At the very least, leaders should consider forming a leadership team for their areas of responsibility. If the leader is a department manager, this may mean a small group of assistant managers or selected employees who work with the manager to provide for the department's leadership function. For example, in the laboratory the leadership team could include the manager, the supervisors of the different functions, and the employee responsible for quality improvement processes or the person who leads the employee governance council. In a nursing inpatient-care department, the leadership team could consist of assistant nurse managers or charge nurses, the department educator, and the manager. The team's purpose determines the membership.

Creating a leadership team within his or her scope of responsibility is a way for the leader to broaden and deepen the leadership strength in the area. It also serves as a tremendous source of support for the leader and improves the leadership thinking and effectiveness. Commitment to decisions made is stronger because there is group ownership and accountability. It can also free up the manager to learn other skills and take a more strategic approach focusing on the issues and challenges of the department or service.

Pitfalls of Creating Teams

This section describes some common pitfalls along the journey in the development of teams.

Often when a team is in trouble, the solution implemented includes the leader giving a pep talk or bringing in a dynamic, charismatic speaker who generates enthusiasm and excitement within the team. This is a quick fix in that the results never seem to last long enough to get the team through the next crisis. More effective in turning the team around is a challenge that creates a sense of urgency. Giving the team a stiff work assignment that team members see as important does more to mobilize stagnated energy and turn it into a productive force than any motivational speech could possibly do.

Not recognizing the special needs and unique challenges based on the type of team is a second common error. Each of the three major types of teams (primary work, ad hoc, and leadership) has unique challenges, and to assume they are all similar is to underestimate the difficulty a particular team may have. For instance, most leadership teams find defining their work and purpose to be problematic. This may seem contradictory because this type of team is composed of leaders who as individuals are usually self-directed and focused clearly on their work. However, most leadership teams confuse their work as a team with the work of the organization as a whole (for example, ensuring the delivery of safe, quality patient care to members of the community versus leading others and creating an empowering environment in which employees deliver safe, high-quality patient care to members of the community).

An ad hoc team formed to lead a change initiative often has difficulty in handing off the project to those who will actually implement it (usually managers) because team members feel a large degree of ownership. This is a basic principle of innovation: the people who implement a change are not as attached to the change as are those who create it. The 1990s produced many examples of this in our health care organizations. Quality improvement initiatives and work-redesign projects in organizations were often designed by people on project teams who then handed off the implementation to managers who did not have the same investment or interest in the project. In most cases, full conversion and implementation failed because no one anticipated this pitfall. Actions can be taken to overcome this difficulty by involving implementers more fully in the process and providing ongoing support during the implementation.

Understanding the unique challenges of each type of team alerts the leader to potential problems. A more complete discussion of these types of teams is available in *Team-Based Health Care Organizations: Blueprint for Success* (Manion, Lorimer, and Leander, 1996).

Ignoring any one of the key elements in creating teams is another major pitfall but one that is relatively easy to correct. For example, a team that had frequent and recurring problems finally called in an external consultant to help. During this work, the consultant discovered that the team had never established members' expectations of one another nor agreed on common working approaches. Simply doing these two things cleared up about 90 percent of the conflicts.

Minimizing the development time to grow a team is common. Too many managers and leaders today believe that if they simply call a group a team, it somehow becomes one. Not taking the time to apply the proper steps of team development often creates a situation in which the group struggles needlessly, trying its best but unable to determine why it's just not working. Unless team members come together to accomplish their work collectively, they do not become a team. Effective teams are those that are emotionally intelligent, able to recognize and process emotion within the group, and regulate themselves in response to daily organizational events. For a team to become emotionally intelligent, it is helpful and perhaps necessary that at least some individual members have a high level of emotional intelligence (Cherniss and Goleman, 2001). However, the mere presence of emotionally intelligent team members does not ensure that the team as an entity will collectively be emotionally intelligent or effective in its performance.

Being able to create high-performing teams is one of the most critical challenges facing leaders today. Virtually every future organizational structure (adhocracy, network, or clustered organization) is based on the premise that teams are to be a prevalent structure. Leaders must have the ability to tap into and release a team's potential. Being able to create successful learning teams is also a strategy identified as effective in dealing with the complexity of open systems.

Leading During Change and Transition

We now turn to the interrelated processes of change and transition. These create significant challenges for leaders. Change today is different: its pace is faster than ever and promises to continue accelerating well into the next decade. The continual onslaught of technological improvements has altered the very nature of work. Service delivery is rapidly shifting from acute hospital care to ambulatory and home care. Health care services are moving from a residency-based to a mobility-based model (Porter-O'Grady and

Malloch, 2003). The rapid rate of mergers and acquisitions in the 1990s resulted in fewer and fewer stand-alone, independent health care organizations. Solutions are shorter lived. The very changes organizations institute to solve problems today may actually become tomorrow's problems. We must realistically view any major change in an organization today as only a stepping-stone to the next change; and these stepping-stones are getting closer and closer together.

Change Versus Transition

Leaders face the challenge of these tumultuous times, and without an understanding of the underlying processes of change and transition, the situation could indeed appear hopeless. The first step for any leader is to clearly differentiate between change and transition. *Change* is an external event that causes an alteration or modification in what has previously existed; *transition* is the internal process that an individual experiences during a psychological adaptation to the change (Bridges, 1991). Transitions take longer than change and may not be evident to others because they are internal. Change is complex, being both a process and an outcome. Leaders effectively lead both.

The Change Process

Understanding change as a developmental process aids the leader in recognizing important sequential steps (Manion, 1993; Manion, Lorimer, and Leander, 1996). We can differentiate five phases, based on an energy model adapted for organizations by organization development consultant Nancy Post (1989). The five phases, illustrated in Figure 5.1, include

1. Preparation
2. Movement
3. Team creativity
4. New reality
5. Integration

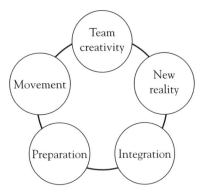

Figure 5.1. A Five-Phase Change Model

Source: From "Chaos or Transformation" by Jo Manion, © 1993, *Journal of Nursing Administration.* Used by permission of the publisher: Lippincott Williams & Wilkins, Baltimore, Md.

Each of these five phases involves several key issues or concerns. Imbalance is created when a key issue is ignored or passed over, or if overemphasis of one issue overshadows the others. Not following the process sequentially results in a prolonged and less effective change process. When a leader understands these five phases and adequately addresses the key issues within each phase, implementing change takes less energy. This model is explained more fully in *Nature's Wisdom in the Workplace: Managing Energy in Today's Health Care Organization* (Cox, Manion, and Miller, 2005).

Phase One: Preparation

The two major issues in this phase include setting the direction and allocating resources. Addressing both of these issues during initiation of a change lays the foundation for a successful effort. In their enthusiasm to begin immediately, many initiators of change pay only scant attention to this stage; once the leader shares the direction, often the leader forgets to review available resources and obtain those necessary for implementation. All issues are equally important.

The leader must examine the purpose of the change. Why is this change needed or appropriate? How will it affect patients, key customers, employees, or the long-term viability of the organization? Will this change help the organization to meet its basic mission? By clearly defining and articulating the purpose of this change, the leader sets the direction for those who will implement it.

Having identified the purpose, the leader considers resources required to implement this change. Although money and financial support are key resources, the lack of other critical resources can be devastating to a change initiative. These other important resources include adequate time; availability of coaches, mentors, and other support people; employees' and managers' skills; and interest from those who must implement the change.

Phase Two: Movement

During this phase, the two primary issues are developing a vision and implementation plan and providing a decision-making structure that enables the project to move forward.

Vision, as described in Chapter Three, is a compelling picture of what the situation will be in the future. A leader's ability to envision a different future, one that is energizing and desirable, makes creating a new reality possible. The most powerful visions are those of a preferred, rather than predicted, future. The envisioned future is a stretch and a challenge. Equally important is the plan that will create this new reality: a specific, concrete, step-by-step plan with time frames and a structure that move the vision from dream to reality.

The leader also determines a decision-making structure at this phase. What is needed to move from idea to concrete change? Is a project team or committee useful? What should the decision-making authority of the people involved be? How does the change affect the present organization or department structure? What measurements or outcomes will determine success?

Phase Three: Team Creativity

This phase is the most dynamic of the five and marks the beginning of actually making the change. Prior to this point, most of the work is preparatory and sometimes considered tedious by enthusiastic and eager leaders. Without the work in the first two phases, however, this phase would not result in lasting change. The four major issues for this phase include coordination and cooperation, the setting of priorities, communication, and climate formation.

Change initiatives fail under the burden of poor coordination and lack of participant cooperation. If coordination is weak, participants may come to believe that the left hand doesn't know what the right hand is doing, which erodes trust and confidence in leadership. During extensive change, those affected are likely to become more egocentric and focused on themselves. Unless leaders are prepared for this phenomenon, they can easily feel anger toward normally cooperative employees and departments that suddenly become obstructive and resistant.

Clearly identifying priorities encourages both leaders and participants to stay focused on the change effort. It is a leadership function to continually evaluate pressing priorities and restate them as often as necessary to help others remain focused on the change. Congruency between leader behavior and stated beliefs is of utmost importance at this time. Because change is difficult and demanding, people implementing a change continually read the signals to ensure that their effort is worthwhile. Leaders must avoid becoming distracted by a new project or the next change, which could cause participants to conclude that the change they are working on is no longer a priority.

Communication is important during all phases of a change initiative, but at this point it becomes critical. A defined communication plan must be conscientiously implemented, including strategies for keeping key stakeholders abreast of changes. Chapter Four includes a more extensive discussion on types and methods of communication.

Creating a corporate culture or climate supportive of the change is essential. If the change requires people to behave in a manner incongruent with the culture, the change is unlikely to succeed.

Phase Four: The New Reality

Once the change has been made and the situation altered, the true impact begins to sink in. Stabilizing the change at this point so that it is anchored for the future and achieving the desired results from the change are the major issues of this phase.

Stabilizing the change is of paramount importance. The leader must execute specific measures to anchor the change into the current reality because without constant pressure, people will revert back to their previous behaviors. Methods for this "include formalizing structures or processes that were used during a trial period, establishing new routines, or formally communicating the new processes to key stakeholders" (Manion, Lorimer, and Leander, 1996, p. 202). An even more powerful method of anchoring the change is to modify the reward system to ensure that the organization reinforces new behaviors. Reward systems include recognition and compensation mechanisms.

The second key issue in phase four is achieving desired results so that the organization regains acceptable productivity levels. Few plans unfold as they were designed. Some planned approaches work, and some do not. Sorting through to find the successful strategies and to eliminate those that are unsuccessful is part of the work of this phase. Leaders must be patient with declining productivity during this trial period.

Phase Five: Integration

Integration is the final phase of the change process, involving review of quality measures, evaluation of results, and management of closure. Unfortunately, it is easy for leaders to undervalue or simply overlook this phase.

The leader now reviews the quality measures identified in phase two, the movement phase. The leader evaluates results and outcomes obtained using these measures to determine the initiative's success. Were desired results achieved? Did any intolerable, undesirable consequences occur? What was the impact on the system, organization, or department? Has quality of service improved? In addition to reviewing quality indicators, the leader should evaluate the actual change process. What organizational learning occurred as a result of this process? How resilient were employees? What leadership skills emerged? How were emotional reactions handled?

The skill with which the leader deals with closure is instrumental in positioning people and the organization well for the next change. "Closure is often the least understood and most often overlooked issue of the entire developmental cycle" (Manion, Lorimer, and Leander, 1996, p. 205). Celebrations are appropriate and help mark the transition occurring. However, closure often includes grief, during which leading others can be difficult. Allowing and supporting any feelings of grief promotes respect for the natural progression of any change and models healthy adaptive behavior.

The Change Process: Five Steps for Success

This five-phase process for implementing change is applicable to change projects of any size. It has guided mergers of hospitals, as well as closures, and been used to implement change in a single department. Understanding the key issues of each phase helps leaders determine progress and prevents common missteps.

Following the phases sequentially reduces the amount of effort and energy that making a change requires. Leaders should read a more thorough explanation of each phase in other sources (Cox, Manion, and Miller, 2005; Manion, 1994; Manion, Lorimer, and Leander, 1996). Too often leaders do not consider key issues, creating major problems later in the process. How many times do organizations embark on changes without enough resources to follow through or without even considering key but less obvious resources such as leadership skill and coaching abilities? How often does a dynamic, charismatic leader grow excited and enthusiastic about a change, exhorting followers to embark on the change without doing necessary preparatory work? How often has everyone been excited about a change, which later did not unfold as planned, with nothing put into place to anchor the change, resulting in one more thing the organization did not follow through on?

The Transition Process

Change alters the way something is done, whereas transition is the psychological adaptation to change. The transition process exists within the change process, but for clarity's sake we address transition here as a separate entity. Bridges (1992) identifies three stages of transition (Figure 5.2):

1. The ending
2. The neutral zone
3. The beginning

Stage One: The Ending

Bridges (1988, 1992) has studied people's reactions to transition for years. He points out that once a leader understands the dynamics of transition, he or she begins to see the need for endings almost

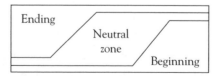

Figure 5.2. Stages of Transition

From *Participant's Guide to Managing Organizational Transitions*, © 1992. Used by permission of the publisher: William Bridges & Associates, Mill Valley, Calif.

everywhere: "Every change in leadership terminates relationships and plans that had been central to people's lives. Every merger takes away power and status that people had built their worlds upon. Every change in product lines or services brings to an end the functions and competencies that made people feel valuable and the groupings that made them feel at home. Even promotions cause people to leave behind their familiar worlds. In short, every change causes loss, whether the change is large or small" (1988, p. 37).

This first stage of transition is painful because it entails saying goodbye to the world one once knew. Valued relationships may end with this change, and individuals lose the comfort of the way things used to be. This stage begins with an awareness that change has forced a closure, a destruction of the known world. This is unsettling—even frightening—to most people.

People in this stage of transition are difficult to work with because they are experiencing the emotions of grief. Anger, irritability, depression, negativism, resistance, and resentment are common during the lowest emotional periods (Manion, 1995). Employees and leaders alike feel vulnerable and out of control. Indeed, in many workplaces expressing anger is not safe because people fear retaliation. When employees are angry with the person to whom they report, this increases their fear.

Stage Two: The Neutral Zone

Once the ending phase is complete, the next stage is the neutral zone. At first glance, this stage seems anything but neutral. It is characterized by disruption, confusion, and fear. "The neutral zone is the psychological in-between time, when it isn't the old way anymore, but it isn't the new way yet either. The old identity is gone but the new identity isn't clear. The old procedures and systems, the old values and norms, the old expectations and priorities are no longer operative or valid, but the new ones haven't taken shape yet" (Bridges, 1992, p. 45).

For most adults, the neutral zone is the most uncomfortable of all transition stages. It can cause tremendous frustration and anxiety because it exists between two worlds, the comfortable known and the frightening unknown. Even if the past was undesirable and fraught with unhappiness, individuals may now romanticize it and remember only its good elements. Compared with the unknown quantity of the future, the past can look pretty rosy. Because the change is in place and the situation has altered, many people assume that internal adaptation will follow at the same pace. Nothing could be further from the truth. Internal adjustment always takes longer.

There is a tremendous urgency in organizations going through change to push people through these first two stages because the characteristic emotions and behaviors are so discouraging. However, without fully experiencing these two stages, transition is not complete; people only suppress the negative feelings. The more repression that occurs, the less likely the organization will achieve the positive, creative side of transition.

Oddly, the second predominant characteristic of the neutral zone is creativity. Because everything is up in the air and uncertain, there is tremendous potential for transforming the way things are done. Chaos and confusion abound, from which creative and innovative ideas arise. "During any period of significant change, one of the leader's most important tasks is to use the change as a challenge to all the assumptions and practices that got the organization to where it is" (Bridges, 1992, p. 51). In times of profound crisis, this challenge reaches to the very core of the organization. What is its mission? How does the organization identify itself? In the face of less significant change, it may simply be an opportunity to ask: Is there a better way to do the things we do?

Stage Three: The Beginning

Bridges (1992) differentiates between the start of something (the change itself) and the new beginning. The beginning implies that people are comfortable with the change and their new identities and that they have rebuilt their world. With a new beginning, comfort and ease have returned; people feel at home again. This is the easiest stage of transition to manage, although it must not be overlooked. At this time, anchoring and stabilizing the change are important.

Pitfalls: Leading Through Change and Transition

Not recognizing the difference between change and transition often leads to ignoring one or the other. Although these two processes are highly interdependent, the value of separating them is to ensure that the leader uses specific interventions to manage each. Change can take place, but when people do not successfully make their transitions and adapt to the change, the change is compromised. People who never adapt to the change have the potential of undermining and destabilizing the change, whether intentionally or inadvertently. In the same way, mismanaged change affects people's ability to successfully adapt to an altered situation.

Examples of this pitfall abound in health care today. Hospitals downsize or merge; organizations implement a patient safety, work-redesign, or continuous process improvement initiative or develop an integrated system—all requiring the shifting or changing of internal organizational culture. But when leaders poorly handle or ignore shaping a new culture and managing people's transition to this new reality, the organization does not gain the full benefit of the initiative. Is it any surprise that the full promise of integration within health care systems has yet to be realized or that most work-redesign and reengineering projects in the 1990s failed?

The most common mistakes in leading change and transition are ignoring the process and rushing people through the stages. Because certain stages result in unpleasant emotions and potentially strained interpersonal relationships, there is a natural desire to pass quickly through these stages or bypass them completely. Although this seems effective in the short term, it only slows the process later.

Less-effective managers and leaders mistakenly believe that managing transition, the people side of change, is a luxury and something too expensive to do. In one organization managers were upset and concerned about the multitude of changes occurring. They believed that their executives were discounting the managers' observations and feelings. When the managers attempted to talk with executive leaders about their concerns, they were told in no uncertain terms that the change was a speed bump and they should just get over it! The managers felt chastised, belittled, and devalued. One would have to question the effectiveness of these executive leaders, because it is the management staff who usually leads the rest of the organization through change. How was this group of executives planning to gain support for the widespread changes after totally and completely alienating this group of people?

Accepting the emotional issues of transition is simply not in the consciousness of the just-get-it-done leaders who are not process oriented. They often ignore the presence of messy emotions and decide they won't let them affect the implementation of change. In the words of one CEO, "I don't want my people being told about these emotions—it's just too negative." Unfortunately, not teaching people what to expect does not prevent the feelings or make the emotions go away. An emotionally intelligent leader recognizes and realizes that emotions, sometimes strong emotions, are part of our workplace environment. To try to separate these emotions from the people who experience them is futile.

During times of change and transition, leaders often exhort people to be more creative, to come up with ideas for dealing with a difficult reality. This can create a no-win situation if the leader is not aware of where employees are in the stage of transition. If employees are trying to cope with closure and are experiencing the emotions of grief, asking them to be creative often results in a demoralizing and self-defeating situation.

Some leaders mistakenly expect these processes to be predictable. Although there is a predictable sequence, no one can accurately forecast the full effects of a change on another person. The change that triggers the emotions of transition may be different for different people. Although one individual may experience a title change as a significant loss, another barely notices. Moving a work space may upset one individual tremendously, but for another, changes in relationships are far more significant.

Conclusion

Exemplary leaders are highly skilled at leading process. They recognize and understand the operative process and are able to guide it in a way that ensures relevant, synergistic outcomes. When process bogs down, they are able to assess the problem, intervene, and redirect the process. Good leaders respect the sequential nature of process and allow it to unfold within its natural time frame. They have the judgment to determine when a process needs a little extra nudge or redirection. Tomorrow's highly effective leader is a master at empowering others, resolving conflict, creating effective teams, and managing change and transition.

Conversation Points

1. Where in your professional life do you see examples of disrespect for process? What is the process involved? What are the consequences of misunderstanding the basic nature of the process?

2. How comfortable are you with facilitating key processes? What are your particular strengths and weaknesses when it comes to being involved in a process? Are you impatient with process, or do you enjoy the challenge? Do you find yourself bogged down, or do you force its closure prematurely?

3. Think of a time when you delegated or transferred responsibility to someone else and the outcome was not what you wanted or expected. What went wrong? Consider the four elements of empowerment (capability, responsibility,

authority, and accountability) and determine where the problem was. What would you do differently today?

4. How do you feel inside when you know a conflict is building and you are going to be involved? What are your physiological reactions? Your emotional reactions? What do you do especially well in dealing with conflict? Where could you improve your skills?

5. What is the most common approach for dealing with conflict in your organization, your department, your life? Is it effective? What are the consequences of these approaches?

6. Think of a time when you used a negotiation process for resolving a conflict. What worked? What were the difficulties? Did you reach a mutually agreeable win-win solution? If not, what happened?

7. Where do teams exist in your organization or department today? Are these teams effective? What was their process for development? Do you have a leadership team in place? How would you go about developing a leadership team for your area of responsibility?

8. Think of changes you have gone through in your organization or department. Did you use a sequential process? What changes were successful, and which changes failed? Why did they fail? How could you use the transition model to facilitate people's transition during changes?

6

Getting Results

*Leaders are proactive—and able to make something
happen under conditions of extreme uncertainty and
urgency.*
    J. W. Kouzes and B. Z. Posner, Encouraging the Heart

Savvy leaders understand that process for the sake of process is not
acceptable. How we achieve results is important; but getting
results, solving problems, and making improvements are ways that
effective leaders do their job and create commitment and credibility
with their followers (Manion, 2004b). And getting results is tightly
connected to the other interpersonal skills this book addresses. For
example, in *Execution: The Discipline of Getting Things Done*, Bossidy
and Charan (2002) report that the first essential skill of getting
things done is to know your people and to continually expand people's capabilities through coaching. This chapter explores several
approaches leaders can use in getting results. It offers a more traditional problem-solving process that is congruent with the quality
improvement processes in many health care organizations today. It
discusses decision making and identifies some common pitfalls. Further, this chapter offers two approaches for tackling tough organizational issues: appreciative inquiry and polarity management.

Problem Solving

In hierarchical, top-down organizations, problem solving is limited in terms of both the people involved and the kinds of problems around which groups meet. Group problem solving is a bottom-up process requiring a visionary leader—a leader who can relinquish control sufficiently to create an environment for employee empowerment. When problem-solving groups are prevalent in an organization, it is a good sign of employee involvement. And knowledgeable leaders understand that it is difficult for individuals to feel empowered if they have no tools with which to solve pressing problems directly affecting their ability to do their work. Seeing improvement in their daily work life creates a sense of momentum and hopefulness for the future in the work group and ensures future participation in these activities. Many quality or process improvement groups are essentially problem-solving groups.

Most effective problem-solving processes include some variation of the following five steps, as outlined in Figure 6.1:

1. Problem identification and analysis

2. A desired future statement

3. Solution generation and analysis of alternatives

4. Action planning and implementation

5. Evaluation

Regardless of what these steps are called, a skilled leader understands that this process must be both sequential and methodical. All steps must be included in the appropriate sequence in order to obtain a quality outcome. Often what passes for problem solving is some spontaneous, inconsistently applied brainstorming technique that follows no proven methodology and misses one or more important steps.

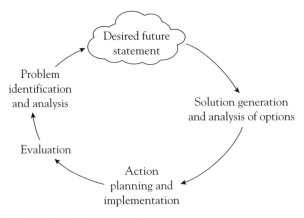

Figure 6.1. A Problem-Solving Process

The following problem-solving process can be effective for either individuals or groups. This discussion will consider group problem solving.

Step One: Problem Identification and Analysis

The group describes and ultimately defines and analyzes the problem. The discussion typically begins with descriptions of symptoms or other evidence of a problem as it affects various members of the group. In many instances, initial statements of the problem are vague and confused. Sometimes the group needs additional information before it can write a problem statement.

It is important to bring to the surface as many characteristics of the problem as possible at this point and to avoid jumping to hasty conclusions. Psychologists who have experimented with thinking for over seventy years have discovered that once a person offers an explanation, he or she has difficulty revising it or dropping it, even in the face of contradictory information. In experiments, subjects were shown an out-of-focus thirty-five-millimeter slide of a fire hydrant. The psychologists found that if a person wrongly identified the object when it was out of focus, he or she often could not identify it when it was brought sufficiently into focus so that another person (who had not seen the blurry slide) could easily recognize it. Their conclusion was significant: more evidence is required to overcome an incorrect hypothesis than to establish a correct one. Individuals who jumped to a hasty conclusion were less sensitive to new ideas and information (Adams, 1986).

Questions often help to define the problem more fully. What are signs and symptoms of this problem? Whom does it affect? Directly or indirectly? How often does it occur? What are all the possible causes or factors involved? The group may determine that it needs more information or data. Many of the techniques taught through quality improvement programs, such as using histograms, fishbone diagrams, pareto charts, and process and scatter diagrams can be helpful at this point (Byers and White, 2004).

During this first step, another important issue to consider is ownership. How have the group or individuals within the group contributed to or created the current problem? This is critical to consider because those alternatives over which the group has control bring a higher rate of success. This is difficult for many groups, who may begin by believing that the fault for the problem lies elsewhere. By pushing themselves, however, they usually begin to see how they have helped create the current situation.

Caregivers in one organization were angry because they often did not have enough clean linen in the morning to complete changing the patients' bed linens. They clearly attributed the problem to the linen services department. When forced to look at their own role in creating the problem, they were clueless. They continued to insist that the other department was at fault. But with persistent prodding, they gradually began to come up with ideas. "We stopped attending the liaison meeting with linen services because we didn't think they were listening to our concerns." They also recalled being told that over $200,000 in scrub clothes were replaced during the year because of employee theft. That money could have helped pay for a higher-capacity washing machine that would process linens faster. The final contributing factor that they identified was their common practice of hoarding linen and stashing it in all kinds of places so that it would be available when needed. This practice had made it impossible to get an accurate inventory count, giving linen services inaccurate figures and thus causing inadequate planning. Once the group identified these issues, it began to work more effectively on the problem. In a radiology department, the problem was inaccurate requisitions for procedures. The radiology employees had contributed to the problem over the years by accepting the patient and doing the procedure in spite of incomplete or inaccurate requisition forms. As a result, there were no consequences for completing (or not completing) the forms.

The problem statement is a concise description of the problem. Novice problem-solving groups tend to put the solution into the problem statement. One group, for example, came up with "The problem is inadequate staffing." Such a statement limits problem-solving creativity because the solution becomes "Get more staff." Changing the problem statement to "There is more work than the current employees can handle" makes multiple possibilities apparent, including eliminating some of the work, changing the way it is being done, and adjusting staffing levels temporarily.

Once the group has clearly identified the problem, the group determines its level of authority in solving the problem (see Chapter Five for a discussion of empowerment). Determining the level of authority at this point is crucial so that everyone's expectations are appropriate. The group can plan necessary communication and involvement with others in the organization. A low level of authority does not preclude a group's working on a particular problem, it simply helps them stay within their scope of authority. And clarity about authority levels will prevent misunderstandings later, when it is time to implement decisions.

Compare the following two groups. Both chose to work on an employee-benefits problem for which they had only level-one authority. The first group was very aware of its level of authority. The members spent their time investigating the problem and gathering information; based on their findings, they made recommendations for the human resource department to consider. Their work focused on a desired future that included the successful presentation of their information and specific steps aimed at their strategies for delivering the recommendations.

The second group had not clarified its level of authority. The members proceeded with enthusiasm throughout the entire process, developing a future vision that included employee benefits, offered in a cafeteria-style approach, from which employees could select. Their action planning revolved around the implementation of the new benefits. They were excited and eager when they finished the problem-solving process, only to become frustrated and angry when the organization did not act on their work. Group members cynically observed that it was the last time they would volunteer for a problem-solving task force, never realizing that the work they had done substantially exceeded their level of authority.

Step Two: Desired Future Statement

A common mistake that problem-solving groups make is to focus almost exclusively on the problem and its causes rather than on what they would like to build or create for the future. Russell Ackoff, the creator of interactive planning, has demonstrated clearly that solutions are more creative if the focus remains on desired outcomes rather than on details of the current problem (Ackoff, Finnel, and Gharajedaghi, 1984).

This step involves asking the question: What would this look like if there were no problem, if it were solved? The group then writes a description of the ideal situation. For example, if the group's problem statement is "Communication between hospital and home health personnel is poor, creating problems in delivery of quality patient care," a desired future statement might be "Communication between hospital and home health personnel is free-flowing, timely, and accurate." In another system a group was working on coordinating community services for seniors. Their desired future statement read: "Community services for seniors are coordinated and easily accessible to participants, with information flowing freely and fluidly between agencies for the benefit of our program participants."

Focusing exclusively on the problem statement leads to more limited solutions. A clear, desirable future statement creates a picture for those involved and generates more imaginative and original ideas, as well as a broader scope of possibilities.

Step Three: Solution Generation and Analysis of Alternatives

This stage is both creative and analytical, and it is critical that the group separate the two phases of this step. The group first generates all possible solutions. It withholds analysis, discussion, and critical thinking about the solutions until it has identified all solutions. Nothing impairs creative flow faster than criticizing or analyzing the ideas as they are presented. Several creativity techniques are useful for generating ideas:

- Nominal group technique

- Mind mapping

- List making

- Attribute analysis

- Storyboards

This section will only briefly describe these, but readers can learn more in the many books available about innovation or creativity (Adams, 1986; von Oech, 1983; von Oech, 1986; Wycoff, 1991).

Nominal Group Technique

This method is often confused with brainstorming, which is unfortunate because most people think of brainstorming as a loose, free-flowing process with few guidelines. Nominal group technique involves a specific process that results in successful outcomes (Del-becq and VandeVen, 1971). The nominal group technique combines quiet, individual thinking time with a structured yet free-flowing sharing of ideas, a technique that is especially useful when group members vary in verbal and other expressive skills.

First, the leader asks a question about the problem, to which group members will individually respond in a specific way. For instance, if the desired future is to have communication between two agencies be free-flowing, timely, and accurate, the leader may solicit responses regarding characteristics required to achieve this state. The group members then individually write down all re-sponses that come to mind after the leader specifies either how many ideas (say, five to ten) each participant should list or the time frame in which to complete the list (perhaps five minutes).

Next, the leader provides these guidelines for sharing the ideas:

Taking turns, every participant gives one idea at a time.

No one is to react in any way to the ideas as they are being pre-sented, which means no clarification or discussion of any kind at this point.

If a group member runs out of ideas, she (or he) can pass until the next turn, when she may present another idea if she has one.

The leader lists each idea on a flip chart or board, with no rewording of the idea, until all the group's ideas are visible. The leader-facilitator then leads a discussion of the ideas to clarify, elab-orate, defend, dispute, or add to the items. The group reviews the list and identifies categories, combining or eliminating some items as needed.

Mind Mapping

This technique is similar to the nominal group process, but the recording of ideas is done in a circular fashion. In a box or oval drawn in the center of the chart or board, the facilitator prints one or two words that capture the essence of the issue. From the previous example, it might be "communication between agencies." As the thoughts and ideas on this topic pour out from the members, the facilitator prints the key words of those thoughts around the essence statement and then connects them to the box with lines. As the group generates ideas that relate to one of those branches, the facilitator prints the idea's key word and attaches it to the branch with a line. Even totally unrelated ideas are captured and printed because they may spark an idea for someone else. Wycoff (1991, p. 48) explains, "Two things happen when you allow yourself to put the idea down—the first is that the mind is freed to go onto other ideas, and the second is that associations are made with this idea. This is where the best ideas come from."

List Making

List making is a commonly used conceptualization technique. It uses the construction of lists as a method of forcing alternative thinking. A simple and effective approach, it starts simply with a question or issue, from which the group members generate a list of ideas to address the subject. The value of list making lies in the fact that checklists require a person to consciously control his or her thinking in order to focus on alternatives that the unconscious mind might ignore in trying to simplify life (Adams, 1986).

Leaders in a head injury rehabilitation center used list making to discover ways of improving the environment for clients (Manion, 1990). Groups of employees were asked to think about things that they would miss or want if a head injury confined them to a rehabilitation facility for the months that recovery would require. Lists were generated and then used to guide changes in the environment at the center. Items generated included the following:

- Pictures of family and friends

- The feel of sun or rain on my face

- The feel of sand between my toes

- The smell of coffee in the morning

- My hair and makeup done every day

- Shopping trips

- Favorite television programs

- Favorite music

- My children staying overnight with me

- Surprises

- Sleeping late in the morning

- Popcorn

- Ability to make my own decisions

- My pets

Attribute Analysis

If problem solvers consider the attributes of a situation, they come to different conclusions than if they operate with generalized stereotyping. Attribute analysis involves breaking the common tendency to generalize. The three steps for this process are the following:

1. List the attributes of the situation.
2. Below each attribute, list as many alternatives as possible.
3. When the list is complete, make many random runs through the alternates, selecting a different one from each column and assembling combinations of entirely new forms of the original subject.

Employees of a new outpatient surgical center wanting to design a user-friendly system with correspondingly friendlier processes used this approach. They began by listing attributes of a user-friendly system: easy access to the building, convenient parking, comfortable waiting facilities for family or friends, speedy admission processes, simplified discharge procedures, a pleasant atmosphere, and procedures scheduled for the client's convenience. They then listed the specific attributes under each of these characteristics. Below convenient parking, for example, they listed "covered, inexpensive or free, safe, and not far from the door or shuttle service."

By listing these various attributes and going through the lists several times in different ways, employees generated several unique approaches that enabled the new center to quickly capture a large segment of the market. These approaches included valet parking, procedures scheduled for the clients' convenience (after-work hours were in high demand), discharge prescriptions available prior to surgery to eliminate a stop at the pharmacy on the way home, comedy videos in the waiting room, beepers to call family members back to the waiting area, and snacks or meals for waiting family members.

Storyboards

Walt Disney created the storyboard as a planning method for his animators (Vance, 1982). It is used to develop and record the creative thinking process. In this context, corkboards or wallboards are used, and cards with ideas are attached to the board. Recording ideas and making them visible often allows us to see the interconnections more easily. One idea often ignites others, and participants can add cards as they come up with ideas. The advantage to using cards is that they can be easily rearranged or discarded. This is a useful technique for stimulating and recording ideas between meetings of the problem-solving group.

One executive team adopted this idea to use during its strategic planning. In developing a group vision, members each received a pad of Post-it notes. The leader asked them to write down one idea per note that described an element of their vision. Individuals generated as many as twenty-five items each. They then shared these and stuck them on large pieces of paper around the room. As the team discussed the notes, categories began emerging, and the leader placed subsequent ideas on appropriate pages. It proved a speedy method of generating and recording a wide assortment of ideas.

The second phase of step three is to analyze all the solutions generated in phase one. Once the group has identified all of the possible alternatives, it can begin to converge regarding the most viable options. A series of helpful questions for sorting and categorizing feasible alternatives include the following:

Are some alternatives very similar? Do they overlap?

Can we combine certain solutions?

Do we need to rearrange any alternatives?

Can we eliminate any? (If yes, do we need to consider any worthwhile applications or characteristics of this option?)

What is good about a solution?

How would it solve the problem or help create the desired future?

Are there any possible unexpected consequences of this option?

If anything goes wrong, what would be the course of action?

What is the group's degree of control or level of authority over this option?

Are there key stakeholders that need to be involved to make this option a success? Are stakeholders likely to support it?

What resources would be needed to implement this solution, and are they obtainable?

Do we need more data and information?

Although this is a lengthy list of questions, each question is important. However, the group needs to think about the answers and get ready to move on. There is no perfect solution for the problems in organizations today, and it is better to implement something than to be caught in a never-ending spiral of data collection. If the selected solution does not work, at least the group has more knowledge and information on which to base a new decision.

At the end of step four, the group should have identified at least two or three viable solutions. Stopping at only one solution is dangerous. If it is not accepted or cannot be implemented, the group members feel demoralized and as though they have wasted their time. Also, research has demonstrated that problem solvers are dominated by pressure to solve the problem and that adopting the first solution may reflect this pressure. Forcing the group to develop at least one alternative results in more creative solutions because group members focus on the desired future as opposed to the need to find an answer.

Deciding among the alternatives requires knowledge of decision-making approaches. There are several types of decision making, including voting and reaching consensus, which this chapter will take up later.

Step Four: Action Planning and Implementation

Determining specific actions to be taken, the time frame within which to complete them, and responsibility assignments for each action must be specific and realistic. Once the group has identified them, it prioritizes the steps to take. In many instances, they must be sequential, because some are dependent on completion of others.

Once the plan is reasonably complete, the group costs out both current practice and recommended alternatives. Spending money or time now in order to save a substantial amount of money or time later can be a compelling incentive to adopt a new practice. In some instances, an alternative can positively affect quality of service without requiring more money. At this stage, the group develops a communication strategy based on who needs to know about this plan and who to include in developing additional expectations. The problem-solving group decides how and when to present its results.

During implementation, one group member must monitor the plan closely to maintain momentum. The group chooses an individual who can also reinstitute the group if further work is necessary.

Step Five: Evaluation

The final step in the problem-solving process is to establish criteria for evaluating success and determine who will be responsible for the evaluations. The parties involved in implementation must know up front how they will measure success. This evaluation criterion should be as precise and objective as possible, which in some instances is fairly simple. A percentage error rate, the number of completed diagnostic tests, the number of patient falls, and figures on employee productivity are a few examples of easily obtained objective measures. Others are more difficult to quantify, such as improvement in relationships between teams or departments, satisfaction levels of key customers, or more subtle changes in the quality of service.

The group establishes specific review dates and makes plans to celebrate the completion of this phase of the group's work. Group members must monitor results and make necessary corrections. Divergence from expected outcomes will mean that the group must identify the cause and find another workable solution. The second and third solution alternatives formulated earlier in the process are helpful in this case. At this point, the leader may need to encourage and remind the group that even if the first recommendation or solution did not work exactly as planned, the solution is now closer than it was before.

This problem-solving process was used effectively in a hospital in the U.S. Sunbelt. An annually recurring problem of a lack of patient beds during the winter months with the influx of visitors from the northern states created conflict between employees and physicians, all scraping to come up with needed resources. Finally, during the summer months, administration initiated a problem-solving team composed of employees, managers, executives, and physicians. This process took several months, but the result was a plan that increased the number of available beds during the winter months and clearly identified backup contingency plans. For the first time in years, the hospital staff managed the winter season without coming to blows over beds.

Pitfalls of the Problem-Solving Process

The most common pitfall occurs when the group does not distinguish when to use problem solving, appreciative inquiry, or yet another approach such as polarity management. This chapter will discuss all these approaches later; all are effective ways of dealing with issues. Some issues are simply better tackled with an approach such as appreciative inquiry; others are not clear-cut problems but polarities to be managed. Determining first which approach to use can prevent a great deal of unnecessary effort.

A second pitfall occurs when the group includes a suggested solution in the problem statement. This limits the variety and creativity of alternatives the group identifies. It comes up with the same old answer one more time. Not only is the solution ineffective, but everyone involved ends up disenchanted.

A third pitfall relates to the group's level of authority. Steps for action must fit the level of authority and the problem. Too often groups develop grandiose action plans that go far beyond their authority and any reasonable parameters. A group of staff working on problems with the employee benefit package when they have no authority to influence the organization's selection or expenditure on benefits is a good example.

Hidden agendas and personal platforms make up the next pitfall. Some group members may have a strategy they want to promote, even if it has little to do with the issue at hand. This cannot be allowed to interfere with a fully explored problem-solving process.

Another common pitfall occurs when the group fails to determine time frames and people responsible for each action step. These are critical to the implementation stage, at which point it is easy for the group to lose steam and neglect to carry out agreed-upon steps. Monitoring and follow-through are essential.

Following the process sequentially is difficult for many groups. The process is a blend of both right- and left-brain activities, and some groups have trouble with one or the other or simply with switching between the two. Problem identification, analysis of alternatives, and selecting action steps and evaluation measures are all examples of logical left-brain thinking. Establishing a desired future and generating all possible options are right-brain thinking, requiring creativity and spontaneity. Groups may facilitate moving from one stage to the other by taking a brief break between them or actually carrying out each step in separate meetings. This creates boundaries between the two types of thinking processes and helps members make the transition. If people in the group are characteristically logical and concrete thinkers, such as clinical laboratory professionals, the group leader may need to be very firm in keeping the group focused during the right-brain activities because the left-brain thinkers will exert tremendous pressure to move to analysis and left-brain logical activities.

Not respecting the problem-solving process as a methodical, sequential process leads to several common problems. The most common is called the Band-Aid approach, often a knee-jerk reaction, when the group moves straight from problem identification to action planning without taking the time to think through a desired future or develop a full range of creative options, as illustrated in Figure 6.2.

Another common problem, called analysis paralysis (Figure 6.3), occurs when the group stays in the problem-identification phase so long that paralysis sets in. The group seems never to have enough data to make a decision; not all the facts have been collected; or there is not enough information with which to move ahead. The goal here is to reach a happy medium between gathering the information and coming to a decision. Collect enough data to provide

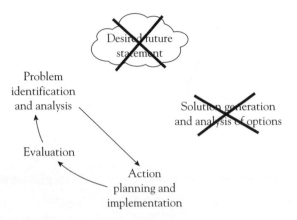

Figure 6.2. The Band-Aid Approach

information for adequate analysis through a specific agreed-upon process and agree to an acceptable time frame for the problem at hand.

Some groups have an exaggerated sense of responsibility and take on too much ownership of the problems. Groups can often avoid this by asking the important question: What is our level of authority for solving this problem? Group members may discover that they do not have an adequate level of authority for implementing a solution to the problem and can therefore accept that doing so is not their responsibility. In some instances, they may realize that they are trying to solve a problem for a key stakeholder not represented and, as a result, modify the membership of their group.

Reasons Groups Bog Down in Process

Both individuals and groups must develop effective problem-solving skills. Most groups process problems rather than solve them, continually discussing the symptoms or effects—anything but the root causes. In many instances, the problem itself escapes discussion, without the group's ever having defined it. Groups engage in unproductive processing for at least three reasons:

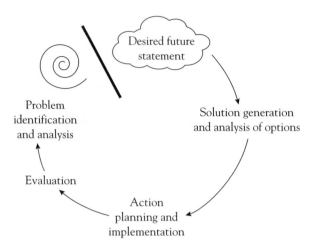

Figure 6.3. Analysis Paralysis

- The group uses voting to determine plans of action, which forces group members to pick sides. Once one person takes a side and another opposes it, the two opposing stances become even more adamant and continue to grow further apart.

- Groups neglect monitoring the group process. Although members may observe an unproductive process, they are too often unwilling to address it. The leader does not ask the nonparticipatory member to contribute, ignores apathy, and tolerates disruptive behavior.

- The group does not recognize or understand its patterns of behavior, which may include closing discussions prematurely or reaching decisions without fully analyzing the problem. Members may not recognize groupthink or behavior that is so polite and courteous that no one dare talk about the real issues. When others do not accept the group's solutions or alternatives, too often the group blames those with authority rather than reviewing its own process and truly evaluating the quality of its work.

Groupthink is a phenomenon "whereby team members become afraid of offering ideas that might conflict with the group's policies and actions. New ideas are often offered weakly and withdrawn quickly if opposed" (Chaleff, 1997, p. 4). Groupthink can destroy creative initiative and even cause people with opposing views to be forced out. The remedy for groupthink is continual self-evaluation of the group's patterns and outcomes.

Leaders who understand problem solving also understand its relationship to decision making. The two are closely interwoven and highly interdependent. Good problem solvers make decisions, and good decision makers use a problem-solving approach.

Decision Making

A *decision*, in this context, is a choice among alternative courses of action that may lead to the desired result. If there are no alternatives, there is no decision to make. Leaders and followers alike assume responsibility for the consequences of their decisions. This can be frightening at times because we make many decisions under conditions of uncertainty.

Decisions are evaluated based on their results or consequences, which are often unpredictable. An individual or group does not have to be right all the time, only most of the time. A sign in a printing shop provided this profound piece of wisdom: "Good decisions come from experience. Experience comes from wisdom. Wisdom comes from making bad decisions." If an individual or group has difficulty dealing with uncertainty, they either postpone decisions until they have resolved all uncertainties or they make poor decisions because they aren't comfortable coping with the uncertainties.

"As important as sound decision-making is, many executives [and groups] neglect to use any formal decision-making process" (Clancy, 2003, p. 343). Good decision makers combine a logical, systematic approach with their intuition. They sort and classify information; differentiate between the valuable, worthless, and redundant; prioritize;

and are able to integrate the whole into an accurate picture of reality. As the amount of information available increases, the complexity of decision making also increases. A leader who is a good decision maker evaluates and recognizes the type of decision the situation calls for. There are at least five types of decisions:

- Individual decisions

- Minority decisions

- Majority decisions

- Consensus decisions

- Unanimous decisions

Individual Decisions

These decisions are made by one person: a leader, a manager or an individual with the responsibility and authority to decide. Others involved are expected to abide by this decision. This type of decision is used when there is no choice; the decision is not important; or the group does not want to make a decision. One example of this is called the "plop," a suggestion that gets accepted without any discussion. Any member of the group can offer the plop.

Individual decisions are sometimes seen as an imposition or a mandated solution directed by someone with the authority to impose such a solution. Impositions are justified when the issue is truly nonnegotiable in terms of responsibility, when a group does not accept responsibility for the solution, or when the decision will have a low impact.

Minority Decisions

Minority decisions occur when a few people or a subgroup of the larger group involved in a situation meet to consider the matter and make a decision. If a group decides that minority decisions are appropriate, the individual or group delegating the responsibility must clearly articulate the expectations for the minority or subset of the group accepting the responsibility. The decision of the minority group is considered binding for everyone involved.

This approach is one that teams and large employee groups often use. A subset of the team examines an issue and makes a decision for the team, which can be a very effective method of decision making when a larger group has difficulty taking the time to navigate the entire process together. It requires a high level of trust within the team or group. Team members with a vested interest in the decision are expected to be part of the subset and are not allowed to later sabotage the decision.

Majority Decisions

When more than half of the people involved in a situation make a decision, it is considered a majority decision and is often referred to as a majority-rules vote. The resulting decision is binding on all. This type of decision is problematic because it may mean that not all members support the result.

A significant disadvantage to majority decision making is that it forces people to take one side or the other. Often the best solutions lie somewhere in the middle. The more firmly one argues for a certain side or solution, the less likely he or she will support an opposing solution if it wins. This form of decision making can be useful when the decisions involve minor issues that do not require 100 percent support to implement or when large numbers of people are involved and no forum or structure exists for resolving minority positions.

Consensus Decisions

A consensus decision results when the entire group or team addresses a problem with all group members, who fully present their views. Consensus exists when each group or team member can honestly make these three statements to every other member (Creative Healthcare Management, 1994):

I believe I understand your point of view.

I believe you understand my point of view.

I believe the decision has been made in an open and fair manner, and I am willing to support the decision whether or not it's my first preference.

In true consensus, no majority-rules voting, bargaining, or averaging of votes is allowed. The process takes more time to achieve but results in active support and prevents sabotage and undermining of decisions. Consensus is especially useful when full team or group commitment to the decision is essential for implementation. In an organization, for example, major decisions such as whether to embark on a major cultural change initiative or to purchase another facility should require the consensus of the entire executive team. If the team makes the decision in any other manner, support may not be present during implementation, when it is required from the entire team.

Unanimous Decisions

In a unanimous decision, each group member fully agrees on the action to be taken, and there is a higher level of commitment. This may be needed when the decision significantly affects each member. A unanimous decision requires 100 percent agreement from group members. Consensus might be described as 70 percent agreement and 100 percent commitment. In other words, the difference between the two is that unanimity requires complete agreement, whereas consensus can be reached with a lower level of agreement. Both result in total commitment.

Group Versus Individual Decisions

Although moving up the decision-making scale from individual to unanimous decisions increases the level of commitment, it also increases the difficulty in arriving at agreement. A leader who is responsible for deciding whether to use individual or group decisions must consider at least five factors:

- *The nature of the problem or task.* Some problems are more easily solved by a group and others by an individual. In creating a new alternative or doing independent tasks, individuals often surpass groups. A project such as creating a new crossword puzzle is best for an individual rather than a group. When tasks are convergent or integrative and require bringing various pieces of information together to produce a solution (such as solving that crossword puzzle), then a group is better. Most goal setting is also more effective in a group because it increases the variety of contributions and level of commitment.

- *The importance of accepting a solution.* When people participate in the process of reaching a decision, they have more commitment to the decision. They work harder and have a greater interest in making the decision successful. When an individual solves a problem or makes a decision, two things must happen: others must be persuaded that this decision is best, and they must agree to act on the decision to carry it out. Not all decisions require commitment, and these can appropriately be made by an individual.

- *The value placed on the quality of the decision.* If a leader is concerned with acceptance of a decision and with empowering others, he or she may accept a decision of somewhat lesser quality because it has widespread acceptance. Decisions that a group makes in the beginning of members' skill development simply may not have the same quality as an experienced individual's decisions. If the quality of the decision is paramount, the group might use an expert in the field.

For example, if a group's members are having communication problems among themselves, they may produce and decide on the problem-solving alternatives to implement. If the outcomes are not beneficial, the group goes back to the drawing board and engages in additional problem solving. Getting it right the first time is not critical. However, if computer hardware problems with a particular application could significantly affect the organization's information systems, a decision to bring in an external expert to solve the problem or make recommendations may be the prudent choice.

• *The characteristics of individual group members.* Effective leaders consider the expertise of the various group members, the stake each has in the outcome, and the role each is likely to play in implementing the decision.

• *The operating effectiveness of the group.* Asking an individual to solve a problem or make a decision may be better than asking a group that is too new to decide or whose members cannot seem to work together. The skills of the group facilitator have an impact as well.

On the upside, group decision making represents greater total knowledge and information. Each group member brings a different perspective, resulting in a greater variety of approaches. Group decisions may have better acceptance and fewer communication problems. Implementation is likely to be smoother and to require less monitoring.

On the downside, a group setting may bring strong social pressure to conform. Groups also tend to err on the side of quick convergence, perhaps settling prematurely on a decision that seems to have support. High-quality ideas introduced late in the discussion have a limited chance of serious consideration. A dominant individual can prevail because of status, verbal skills, or persistence. Hidden agendas create problems in group decision making. Unless the leader brings these to the surface, they result in skewed and sometimes unfair or poor decisions. A significant problem for group decision making is that it simply takes longer for a group to decide.

Pitfalls of Decision Making

The most common decision-making pitfall is approaching decisions without due consideration of the various types of decision making. Without carefully analyzing the situation or giving sufficient thought to outcomes, a leader may miss opportunities for effectively engaging others in the decision. Followers can fall into the same trap. There are appropriate occasions for all types of decision making, but if followers expect to participate and reach consensus and the leader is making an individual decision, the group will not meet followers' expectations.

In one urgent-care business, Ellen, the CEO, decided to reorganize and restructure the leadership and management ranks. Several managers were furious because Ellen did not include them in any discussion but instead simply told them what the new structure would be. Ellen elected to make an individual decision, which was her right as CEO. Unfortunately, however, she had been preaching empowerment for some months, and those committed to empowerment in the company saw her individual decision as a slap in the face. An open discussion about how decisions would be made and which were to be individual and which were to be group decisions might have prevented some of these hard feelings.

The second common pitfall is a lack of understanding of consensus. *Consensus* has become an overused and misused buzzword in recent years. Some people mistake participatory decision making (in which the leader gets input from members but a small group or an individual actually makes the decision) as consensus. Consensus is first and foremost a *group* decision-making process. If a decision truly needs to be made by consensus, no one should assume that the group has met the conditions of mutual belief, understanding, and support. Because reticent or disagreeing group members may not come forward or openly oppose the decision, the leader needs to actually ask each member of the group to state his or her commitment to the decision.

As an example, a statewide ad hoc committee, whose task it was to recommend a new organizational structure for the state hospital association, spent long hours debating this hot political issue. When the group finally settled on a recommendation, the leader asked for consensus. The leader individually asked every group member the following three questions: "Do you believe you understood everyone else's point of view? Do you believe your point of view was fully expressed and understood by the others? Can you support this decision?" Each stated his or her agreement. At the annual meeting, however, one of the committee members had second thoughts when realizing members from a special interest group of which he was also a member were upset about the committee's final recommendation. This member began talking with key association members, trying to engender support for an alternative and basically undermining the committee's work. During a public discussion of the issue, the leader reminded association members that they had reached the recommendation by consensus and reviewed exactly what *consensus* means. When reminded that he had agreed to support the committee's decision, the individual ceased his efforts to overturn the recommendations.

Not carefully considering the various factors in group versus individual decision making can be a major pitfall for a leader. A healthy combination of the two is important. In some instances, explaining why the group will use one or the other is also appropriate.

Decision making is closely related to problem solving but involves its own special issues. Exemplary leaders are good decision makers, but they also are able to relinquish control and engage others in decision making when circumstances warrant. Shared decision making can strengthen any organization as long as it follows careful consideration. Understanding and applying the four key concepts of empowerment (capability, responsibility, authority, and accountability) can help make shared decision making successful.

Appreciative Inquiry

An alternative approach to traditional problem-solving or process improvement methodology is a form of action research known as appreciative inquiry. It is based on the belief that something is already working well in the organization. Finding it and studying it can lead to not only a deeper understanding but insight into how to overcome the current difficulties and design a more desirable future.

The research world knows well that what we dwell on increases in our life. It follows that focusing on problems simply brings more problems or difficulties. To appreciate something suggests that we hold it as positive; we see the positive traits or characteristics; and this increases its value, much as a home appreciates in value over the years. Appreciative inquiry is based on generative learning: "an ability to see radical possibilities beyond the boundaries of problems as they present themselves in conventional terms. High-performing organizations that engage in generative, innovative learning are competent at appreciating potential and possibility. They surpass the limitations of apparently 'reasonable' solutions and consider rich possibilities not foreseeable within conventional analysis" (Barrett, 1995, p. 2).

Comparing Traditional Problem Solving and Appreciative Inquiry

Traditional problem solving often involves looking back at our failures and trying to discover the causes. Appreciative inquiry instead involves inquiring into our successes so that we can discover the distinctive attributes we can use to build on performance and create new strategic approaches. Traditional problem solving is a more mechanized approach based on the belief that problems can be isolated, broken down into separate parts, repaired, and then restored to wholeness. As an approach, it often totally misses the systems implications. And just as one can dissect the body and learn about it even at the smallest cellular level, we have yet to discover the true essence of the person, the soul or the personality, that really makes each of us who we are. In the same way, problem solving often misses the essence of a situation.

Problem solving is likely to be more effective in dealing with issues that are more oriented toward process improvement, such as inaccurate radiology requisitions or extended waiting time for patients in the emergency department. Appreciative inquiry works well for issues related to less logical and methodical processes, such as changing the work culture. In some instances, a major issue might include both approaches. Reducing patients' waiting times in the emergency department is an example of an issue that has both specific process improvement opportunities as well as needed cultural changes.

Proponents of appreciative inquiry point out that a problem-solving approach has many consequences, including the following:

- *It limits the approach to the issue.* Often we accept the constraints of the status quo, which leads to coping with a problem rather than fixing its cause. Take, for example, the problem of a very high patient census and the potential need for diverting patients from the emergency department to another local facility. Employees in one hospital were asked what they would do if the city's other emergency department was also diverting patients. They were stymied and could come up with no solutions. When asked about setting a limit on elective admissions to ensure that beds were available for emergency admissions, they found this inconceivable because they felt administration would never consider such an approach. Yet it *is* a solution, just not a popular one. And until the organization does something to create a different scenario for these people, all of their planning is based on coping with an untenable situation. At what point does it become riskier to continue to admit patients when there are not enough resources to provide for their safe care? This example simply illustrates the difficulties inherent in using a mechanistic problem-solving approach.

- *It creates an orientation toward finding deficiency.* The assumption is that something must be wrong somewhere. Managers develop self-worth as problem solvers, and so do executives. Thus, the more problems, the more important these people are! This can lead to the dysfunctional behavior of stirring the pot, creating problems in order to step in to solve them.

- *It creates a fragmented view of the world.* People in the organization become more and more expert in smaller parts of the system. Along the way it is easy to lose our ability to see the system as a whole and to understand the interdependencies and the intricate connections that exist.

Ludema, Cooperrider, and Barrett (2000, p. 8) sum up the consequences of an organizational focus on problem solving quite well: "As people in organizations inquire into their weaknesses and deficiencies, they gain an expert knowledge of what is 'wrong' with their organizations, and they may even become proficient problem-solvers, but they do not strengthen their collective capacity to imagine and build better futures."

In health care today, one of the most important organizational tasks is the creation of learning cultures (Tichy, with Cardwell, 2002). An appreciative learning culture allows employees to explore, extend their capabilities, and experiment at the very margins of their expertise and knowledge. This all serves to improve our ability to meet our mission—high quality care for patients and clients.

The Appreciative Inquiry Process

Although there is no cookie-cutter approach to appreciative inquiry, scholars have identified several general principles and stages. One of the most important principles is to form a positive question or statement of the topic. This is the most critical part of the entire process because it serves as an intervention in and of itself (Zemke, 1999). And although it sounds easy enough to accomplish, in truth, most people who are faced with a difficult issue or challenge to deal with tend to focus on the negative and to create a problem-oriented question. Take, for example, the need to improve physician and employee interpersonal relationships and communication. The tendency is to identify this issue as a "need to improve physician-employee working relationships." This statement implies that something is currently wrong, and it carries with it complex baggage such as the unequal positional power of physicians and employees or the difference between employees and independent practitioners.

The challenge is to create questions that "inspire and encourage people to give . . . positive examples to use as models" (Zemke, 1999, p. 29). A leader might say: Give me examples of positive working relationships between employees and physicians. One could further explore the characteristics of these relationships: What makes these relationships work so well? Another approach would be to say: Describe what it is like when you have a good working relationship with a physician (or with an employee). If the topic is not affirmative, the initiative will fail.

Stages of Appreciative Inquiry

The stages of appreciative inquiry are discovery, dreaming, design, and destiny (Figure 6.4).

Discovery

This is often referred to as the appreciating phase, and it involves storytelling. It is a very collaborative stage. Participants think of examples and experiences that illustrate or answer the appreciative

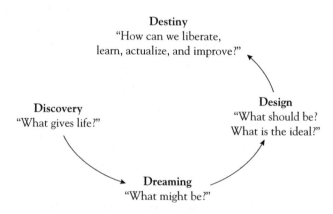

Figure 6.4. Stages of Appreciative Inquiry

question and share them. They focus on those moments of excellence and identify the factors and characteristics that made them possible. This stage basically answers the question: What gives life? From this work, it is possible to build consensus around the strengths or basic principles inherent in the issue.

As an example, one organization was concerned about creating a more positive work environment in order to attract and better retain employees. The leader used an appreciative inquiry approach. These were questions from this first stage: Think of a time when you felt most energized and alive at work. What was happening? Who was there? Describe the workplace environment. Some of the answers included the following:

- I felt valued.

- I was learning a new skill.

- My manager coached me so I could build my expertise.

- I was involved in helping make the decision.

- There was progress as a result of our actions.

- What I did made a difference.

- I liked the people I was working with.

- We had a great team.

- I was asked my opinion and it was used in making the final decision.

- I had a high level of autonomy.

From this first step, the group developed a list of positive attributes that described these environments.

Dreaming

The second stage is the dreaming stage, also known as the envisioning phase. The basic question is: What might be? This stage often starts off with an exercise such as this: "Let's assume that tonight we fall asleep and wake up five years from now. When you wake up, the hospital has become exactly the organization you would like it to be. What do you see that is different and how do you know it is different?" (Zemke, 1999, p. 30). The result of this stage is that the group coalesces around a vision for the group or the organization and drafts a statement of what it will look like in the future. Based on the previous example, a vision statement might be something like: "Our workplace environment is one in which there are healthy working relationships between people, there is a high level of employee involvement in decision making, and people are treated with respect and valued for their contribution."

This stage is similar to the visioning approach presented in Chapter Three. It is not merely a dream but a vision that is grounded in history, tradition, and facts. It is based on examples of what has worked.

Design

This is also referred to as the co-constructing phase because the work is to design the ideal. The questions here are: What should be? What is the ideal? What are the principles that will help translate this vision into action? How can we make this happen? Many successful books in the business literature use this approach. Interested individuals carefully study successful organizations or businesses to determine the principles that led to their success and then, as authors, share them with others who attempt to emulate them.

A disadvantage of trying to duplicate another organization's successes is the resistance one often encounters because "no other organization or business is exactly like ours." People often use the differences as explanations for why a change cannot happen. One of the advantages of using an appreciative inquiry approach within the organization is that it takes away this rationalization or excuse. If this positive environment can be created in the imaging department, why not in the laboratory department? After all, similar financial constraints exist; the medical staff is basically the same; the community issues are shared; and so on.

Destiny

The destiny phase is also known as the sustaining phase. The question is: How can we liberate, learn, actualize, and improve? The participants focus on how to actualize, sustain, or create these characteristics. Zemke (1999) notes that originally this stage stood for delivery; the work was focused on developing action plans, building implementation strategies, and monitoring outcomes. Cooperrider and his colleagues (Zemke, 1999) have greatly deemphasized this concrete work in favor of more spontaneous, free-form activities. Simply preparing people in the organization with the process of the first three steps and then letting them apply them on their own in the organization has been successful in many different types of businesses around the world.

The end result of an appreciative inquiry process depends on the topic that started the cycle. It may be a culture change or the development of a vision and plan to put into place.

Polarity Management

There is yet another approach to dealing with challenges in getting our work accomplished. In some instances, the issue or difficulty we are dealing with is not a problem as such but rather what Barry Johnson (1996, p. xviii) calls a polarity: "Polarities are sets of opposites which can't function well independently. Because the two sides of a polarity are interdependent, you cannot choose one as a solution and neglect the other." Believing that everything we face is a problem results in trying to solve some problems that are simply unsolvable,

even with all the necessary resources. By seeing polarities as problems to solve, we greatly undermine ourselves, wasting time in futile
efforts. There are many examples of polarities in health care organizations today:

The need for leadership versus management skills

Emphasis on individual effort versus team initiative

Coaching others to do difficult things versus the manager doing them

Management accessibility and visibility versus management
think time and privacy

Rigidity in implementation of policies versus flexibility

Priority on employee needs versus patient needs

Service at any cost versus cost-effectiveness and wise use of
resources

Commitment versus compliance

Specialization versus generalization of employees and physicians

Centralization versus decentralization of services

If we see any of these polarities as problems to be solved, we waste
our efforts. There are no clear-cut solutions to these issues.

Johnson's approach (1996) involves identifying when the issue
is actually a polarity and managing it as such, rather than treating
the situation as a problem to be solved. "The objective of polarity
management is to get the best of both opposites while avoiding the
limits of each" (p. xviii). In other words, the manager has the judgment to reward both individual and team effort and understands
that any modern organizational system not only has room for both
models but needs both. In some instances, an individual can best
carry out the work, whereas in other situations, a team is much
more effective. Overemphasis on either end of the polarity can
result in problems.

The way to manage a polarity, Johnson (1996) suggests, is through using a grid or polarity map with two poles (Figure 6.5). The left half represents one side of the polarity, and the right half represents the other. The upper half represents the positive outcomes that focus on the particular pole, and the lower half represents the negative outcomes that come from focusing only on that pole. Before you can effectively manage a polarity, you have to be able to see all four quadrants of this polarity grid. Johnson suggests filling out whichever quadrants are easiest first and then working from there.

Figures 6.6 and 6.7 show polarity maps that represent the four quadrants of an issue that a respiratory care department in a large tertiary medical center faced. The pediatric respiratory therapists included those who worked in general pediatrics and others in the neonatal intensive care unit. Conflict arose periodically over the years

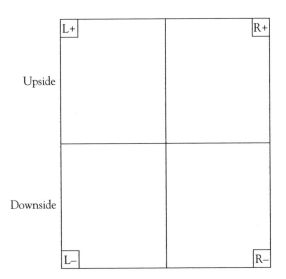

Figure 6.5. The Polarity Map

Source: From *Polarity Management: Identifying and Managing Unsolvable Problems,* by Barry Johnson, © 1992, 1996. Used by permission of the publisher: HRD Press, Inc., Amherst, Mass., www.hrdpress.com.

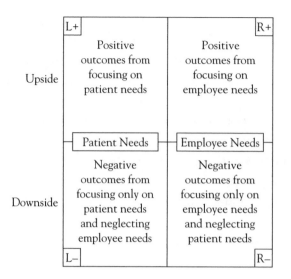

Figure 6.6. Polarity Map: Patient Needs Versus Employee Needs

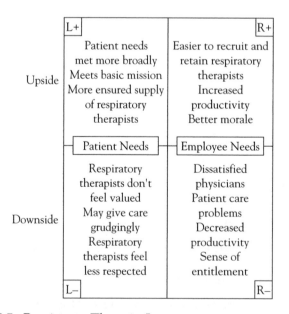

Figure 6.7. Respiratory Therapist Issue:
Putting Patient Needs or Employee Needs First?

about the issue of specialization versus generalization of these practitioners. The neonatologists and pediatricians were often in direct conflict with each other as well as the manager of the department about the issue. When the manager facilitated the group examining this as a polarity, they identified the underlying issue as determining whether patient needs or employee needs are paramount.

Mapping out this polarity enables you to see the whole picture or structure of the dilemma. To focus exclusively on patient needs may result in not meeting important employee needs, which may then result in lower morale and productivity, indirectly affecting how the respiratory therapists meet patient needs. The clearest opposites in the polarity map are the downside of one polarity and the upside of the other. Johnson (1996, p. 11) calls movement through the grid the "Polarity Two-Step." It starts in either lower quadrant and moves across and up, down, and then repeats.

The difficulty in dealing with polarities occurs because each party is convinced that it is right in its particular conviction and basically sees only its side. Working the group through the polarity map helps create the whole picture. Instead of the parties disagreeing and contradicting each other's view, the task becomes to supplement each other's view in order to see the entire picture. Parties on both sides of the polarity have key pieces to the puzzle; they just need this simple structure to help identify and share them. The opposition that each side feels to the other actually becomes a key resource in dealing with the issue. No one is being challenged; instead, both parties assume the accuracy of each position. As a result, there is joint effort in combining two valid views of a situation in order to see a more complete picture.

Johnson (1996, p. 45) says that "in most organizations there are often very serious and costly confrontations that take place because a 'both/and' polarity is treated like an 'either/or' problem to solve." In working out the polarity map together, the possibility of each participant seeing the other quadrants and more fully understanding the issue occurs because the process has not contradicted their own view of reality but confirmed it. "Successful management of polarities calls for intentional interventions that support both values (poles) simultaneously" (Wesorick, 2002, p. 24).

One of the difficult challenges is knowing when there is a polarity to manage instead of a problem to solve. Johnson (1996) offers two questions to use for help in deciding which you are facing: (1) Is the difficulty ongoing? (2) Are there two interdependent poles?

If a solution exists that is a definite end point in a process, the problem is solvable. Take for example, the decision about where to have the holiday party. Once the group makes the decision, it is done. This is an either-or problem: either we go here or we go there. Once the group makes the decision, it is carried out. Problems of choice are solved the minute the choice is made. But solving polarities, on the other hand, is a continual process. Instead of reaching an end point, there is a never-ending change of emphasis or focus from one pole to another. For example, emphasizing and rewarding individual performance is appropriate at some times, and focusing on the team effort is appropriate at other times.

The second question is whether there are two poles that are interdependent. "The solution in problems to solve can stand alone. Unlike a polarity to be managed, the solution to a problem to solve does not have the necessary opposite that is required for the solution to work over an extended period of time" (Johnson, 1996, p. 82). Polarities instead require both poles. The issue of manager accessibility to employees is an example. On the one hand, for the manager to be available to employees is an important aspect of the job; yet the manager also needs to have quiet, uninterrupted time in order to do the work that requires concentrated thinking time.

Once the polarity map is complete, the question is: What do we need to do to stay in the upper two quadrants? In the respiratory therapist example, the question is: How can we meet both patient and employee needs? How do we know when to shift the focus from one pole to another? The group then has identified actions to support each side of the polarity and is more likely to recognize in the future when overemphasis on either pole has occurred.

Conclusion

This chapter has focused on results and several key processes that effective leaders use in obtaining results, specifically the skills of problem solving and decision making. Two additional approaches are included to broaden the leader's repertoire, appreciative inquiry and polarity management. These skills, combined with the interpersonal skills that previous chapters delineated, increase the leader's ability and credibility.

Conversation Points

1. What typical system or department problems do you deal with currently? How effective are problem-solving groups in your department or organization? What process do they use?

2. Think of the different types of decision making (majority vote, consensus, individual, and so on) and identify examples of each that you see in your work environment.

3. Are you better with right-brain (spontaneous, creative, free-flowing) thinking or left-brain (logical, analytical, and methodical) thinking? What about your work group? What is the impact on the effectiveness of your problem-solving efforts?

4. How could you use appreciative inquiry to deal with issues you are facing?

5. What common polarities do you see in your workplace? Have they been mistaken for problems? How could you use the polarity grid to achieve more effective results?

7

Developing Others

Managers who see themselves as coaches will also tend to see their employees as individuals of innate talent and worth.

Ron Zemke, *"The Corporate Coach"*

Leadership is the art of influence, the capacity to move or impel others to a certain course of action. Each competency explored in this book increases the leader's ability to influence others. A healthy, vibrant relationship with followers is the foundation for exemplary leadership (see Chapter Two). Shared values, a strong sense of purpose, and clarity of vision build commitment to a common direction. Free-flowing, consistent, and accurate communication between leaders and followers directly affects leaders' influential abilities. Skill at leading processes and getting results are additional competencies (see Chapters Five and Six). A final manner in which leaders influence is by helping followers develop their skills and abilities.

The Leader's Role

Developing others is the final leadership competency this book addresses. One might argue that an effective leader, accomplished in the other skills already presented, spontaneously and involuntarily helps others develop. People simply observing the leader's behavior are influenced by it. Most leaders, however, are not content with a passive role in developing others and instead choose an intentional path that actively focuses on supporting the evolution of followers into leaders. The intentional development of others is the focus of this chapter.

The intentional development of people in the organization is a strategic focus, a future-oriented strategy that exemplifies hope and optimism. Tichy and Cardwell (2002) believe that winning organizations are successful precisely because they have leaders at all levels; and they have leaders at all levels because they make the development of internal leaders a priority. They point out that the top leaders "personally devote enormous amounts of time and energy to teaching, and they encourage other leaders in the company to do the same" (p. 3).

This chapter will thoroughly explore the methods of coaching for performance improvement, providing opportunities, and teaching. The chapter will further identify approaches that increase the leader's effectiveness and delineate a specific coaching process. All are based on the premise that the leader's influence on others increases if the leader engages actively in the process of developing followers.

Coaching

Today's leadership rhetoric is filled with references to coaching. Writers exhort leaders and managers to become coaches; articles and books on coaching in the workplace appear regularly; and seminars on the topic are selling out. With this insistent and repetitive urging to become a coach, why aren't more leaders excellent coaches?

The good news is that through years of experience and learning, some leaders and managers do develop excellent coaching skills. However, they may not have a concrete framework that is easy to pass along to others because they learned their skill over years of practice, trial and error, and careful scrutiny of what worked and what did not. Excellent coaches with years of experience acquire intuition, a sense of knowing something without understanding how one knows it. Coaching becomes a consistent and vital part of their leadership practice because they have directly observed and received its many benefits. These health care leaders continually seek to further refine and define their coaching role. What exactly does *coaching* mean? What do I do as a coach for my followers?

Now the bad news: many health care managers and leaders engage in a passive form of coaching, characterized predominantly by inconsistent and sporadic coaching. On one project, they take an active coaching role, only to have followers accuse them of micromanaging; and on another project, they offer little or no guidance or advice because they are too busy. Perhaps the only consistent behaviors are the annual performance appraisals and disciplinary processes meant to address and correct performance problems. This is a reactive rather than a proactive process—often something that leaders dread rather than see as an integral part of their role.

Unfortunately, the bad-news description is more common in today's workplace. According to Ron Zemke (1996, pp. 26, 27), "Given the growing popularity of the coaching metaphor and the facility with which it slips from the lips of consultants and managers alike, you might expect by now that most managers would excel at listening, setting a positive example, giving praise, pointing out areas of improvement, and encouraging employees to stretch and grow—the skills of coaching. Naturally you'd be wrong." He goes on to report on recent studies, all of which conclude that "on a wide range of skills, managers were rated lowest in their ability to give employees useful feedback on job performance."

Why Leaders Don't Coach

If coaching is so important and popular today, why is it so rare? Why is it inconsistently practiced? Why is there aversion to functioning as a coach? There are many possible reasons.

Lack of Understanding

Leaders know that coaching followers for performance improvement is important. After all, isn't everyone telling them so? Some leaders are ineffective coaches because they do not understand the principles involved; they may never have received coaching themselves and so have no role models from whom to learn. When leaders are managers and part of the organizational hierarchy, managerial responsibilities further cloud the issue. Some believe that completing performance appraisals on time means their coaching responsibilities are over for the year. There is confusion over the difference between counseling and coaching. *Counseling,* as Minor (1989, p. 2) defines it, is "a supportive process by a manager to help an employee define and work through personal problems that affect job performance." Coaching is defined later in this chapter.

Lack of Time

Downsizing and restructuring in health care organizations have taken their toll in terms of formal leadership positions. Leaders with hierarchical positions have more responsibility and broader spans of control than ever. The rapidly accelerating pace of change places many additional time demands on today's leaders and can easily result in physical and mental exhaustion. Unfortunately, coaching is a leadership function that is easy to put off. Finding time to coach just does not feel like a priority when a leader is already facing a full and frenetically busy day. Good leaders understand that coaching is an investment for the future. It takes time now but later returns huge dividends.

Fear of Confrontation

Addressing performance gaps sometimes feels like confrontation, especially if the performer receives the comments less than graciously. A leader's reluctance to correct or suggest alternative approaches creates a downward spiral. Afraid of offending the person or precipitating an emotionally negative response, the leader delays giving the person much-needed performance feedback. The leader becomes increasingly conscious of the performance gap and with every occurrence comes to believe more and more strongly that he or she must address it. Reluctance fuels procrastination, and when the leader and performer finally discuss it, the simple performance gap has become a major issue. When the leader and follower both clearly understand the purpose of coaching and the leader addresses the issue immediately, performance feedback does not assume horrific proportions.

Lack of Confidence

Coaching skills are learnable, but trial-and-error experience can be painful. Classroom time on coaching rarely goes beyond theory. Although being coached is one of the best ways to learn coaching, leaders who have not received coaching themselves feel they are fumbling through the process. And they may even be coaching followers who are more highly competent in a particular area than they are, so it is no surprise that the leader's confidence may waver and weaken.

Lack of Incentive

Little in today's organization incites leaders to develop others. One department manager noted that when he worked hard to develop people within his department, they were promoted to positions elsewhere in the organization. Initially, he was pleased and satisfied by this because he believed this was his role as a leader. Over time he realized that an employee's promotion left him with a major deficit in his department and the need to start the process all over again—finding the right employee and pouring time and effort into guiding the new employee's development. As a fully mature manager-leader, he continues to engage actively in this process, though he admits he is tired after several decades of this cycle. How different he would feel, he has mused, if the organization would give him a $10,000 bonus for every employee it promoted outside of his department! Successfully recruiting an external applicant for a position often costs far more than that, so both he and the organization would conceivably come out ahead. And if a personal bonus is not feasible, an incentive in the form of money could go to his department with the freedom to use it as he and his work group decide.

These reasons all offer some explanation for the lack of active coaching in today's health care organizations. Admittedly, the good news–bad news scenario is more likely a continuum with each at opposite ends. More leaders and managers are likely to fit somewhere in the middle than in the extremes. This chapter section defines coaching and proposes a concrete process that creates a structure to help make the coaching process easier to engage and apply in day-to-day work.

Coaching Defined

Coaching has become a buzzword in health care leadership circles. Buzzword status is dangerous because the term becomes so commonly used in a superficial manner that it often becomes meaningless. Instead of frequent use increasing understanding, the opposite occurs. Examples of familiar buzzwords include *empowerment, paradigm,* and *team.*

Webster's describes *coach* as a verb meaning "to give instruction or advice." It further defines it in terms of sports and the arts but makes no mention of the coach in the business or work world. This chapter will define coaching as a process of facilitating an individual's or team's development through giving advice and instruction; encouraging discovery through guided discussions and hands-on experiences; observing performance; and giving honest, direct, and immediate feedback. Coaches ask questions to stimulate discovery and thinking on the part of the follower. The goal of coaching is to improve the individual's or team's skills and abilities. Don Shula (Shula and Blanchard, 1995, p. 28), longtime coach of the Miami Dolphins, says, "A good coach provides the direction and concentration for performers'

energies, helping channel all their efforts toward a single desired outcome. Without that critical influence, the best achievements of the
most talented performers can lack the momentum and drive that
make a group of individuals into champions."

It is helpful to distinguish between the process of coaching and
the role of coach. As a process, coaching refers to the way outcomes
are achieved. It includes the procedure or structure applied in order
to obtain desired results. In the definition, for instance, giving advice
and instruction is one way that the desired outcome—facilitating
the individual's development—is realized. In this instance, *to coach* is
an action, an active verb.

Coach is also a term used to describe a position or role that a person takes on. The coach is an individual who applies a process of
coaching. This implies some level of formal structure, for every position or role carries responsibilities. The level of formality in the relationship can range from contractual (a legal agreement defining
the role and relationship of coach to the individual receiving the
coaching), with everything clearly spelled out, to a loose agreement
whose details are implied by the participants involved.

In today's workplace the structure tends to be on the loose to
the nonexistent side. A leader or manager may intellectually know,
and even accept, that coaching is an important function of his or
her role yet engage in the process only sporadically and reactively,
with actual coaching occurring when the leader delegates new tasks
and responsibilities or when performance shortfalls are apparent.
Formalizing the coaching relationship to some degree may provide
a structure that converts an inconsistent and reactive process to one
that is consistent and proactive.

The Coaching Role

Comparing the coaching roles of health care leaders to athletic
coaches sheds light on the concept. There are many similarities,
although there are also some striking differences, such as this major

one: most individuals on a sports team are highly motivated to be there—not always the case in the workplace. Similarities in these different arenas, however, are striking: the coach recruits and selects players, determines the game plan, works with the team to improve performance by giving feedback, continually evaluates the team's performance, and motivates and encourages the team or the individual.

In health care organizations, as in sports, the coach does not have to be a star player—not always the best criterion for a good coach. The coach must know enough about what he or she is coaching to make suggestions that are to the point and helpful. But primarily the coach is highly skilled at helping others do better. Without the coach's objective viewpoint, a performer may repeat the same mistake over and over again. Yet often in health care settings, employees expect the leader to be the expert or star in clinical skills; indeed, many leaders have come to expect this of themselves.

In sports, the coach would not dream of missing a game or not being present when the team practices or competes. Yet many leaders in health care are so inundated with paperwork and meetings that they coach primarily by voice and e-mail, spending little time actually observing performers at work. "Coaching is an intensely personal business. You can't coach people from a distance, with aloofness. People need to see that you are at least as interested as they are in what's going on" (Shula and Blanchard, 1995, p. 125).

Another important point from the sports world helps health care leaders understand their coaching role. In sports, it would be ludicrous for star players not to work with a coach. Yet in a health care setting, too often the focus of the manager is on poor performers, to the neglect of exemplary performers. Because the exceptional employee is not creating any problems, the coach may believe that he or she would better spend time with low performers. Yet the future yield from investing in good employees is dramatically higher than focusing all efforts on those at the lower end of the performance continuum.

Sports analogies may induce visions of competition, one team winning over another. In this regard, the health care leader–coach may be more like a theater or movie director, a symphony conductor, or a dance coach. These coaches function in much the same way as a sports coach, but the desired outcome is one that is mutually beneficial for all rather than victory in a win-lose competition.

Before presenting a process for effective coaching, we must address at least two general principles or concepts that provide a grounding in the basic theory. The first relates to the formation of a relationship between coach and performer, and the second is the application of the principles of motivation.

Building the Relationship

A prerequisite to effective application of a coaching process is the establishment of a relationship between coach and performer or player. Coaching, much like leadership, simply cannot exist in the absence of a relationship. Its very essence is interaction between people. And without a sound relationship, the performer is simply unwilling to act on the advice and counsel the coach shares, as established by principles presented in Chapter Two. The presence of a relationship characterized by trust, mutual respect, and open communication (discussed at length in Chapters Two and Four) greatly influences the quality of a coaching relationship.

Trust

Trust, the foundation, comprises the three elements of competence, congruity, and constancy. A coach who knows the rules of the game and has established his or her own competency can be an excellent coach without ever having reached star status based on his or her own performance. In fact, some star players who have gone on to be coaches have failed dismally because good coaching takes far more than expert performance skills. More important are adequate knowledge of the game and expert coaching skills.

The second element of trust—congruity—enhances faith and is heightened when the coach behaves in a manner that matches the message that the coach is sending the performer. Successful sports coaches understand this concept. In discussing reasons for the phenomenal success of his teams, Don Shula, long-time successful coach of the Miami Dolphins, writes (Shula and Blanchard, 1995, p. 56):

> A lot of leaders want to tell people what to do, but they don't provide the example. "Do as I say, not as I do," doesn't cut it. Of course, I'm not about to show players how to run or pass or block or tackle by doing these things myself. My example is in things like my high standards of performance, my attention to detail, and, above all, how hard I work. In these respects, I never ask my players to do more than I am willing to do. My own preparation for every game has to be exemplary. I am dedicated to success and will do whatever it takes to achieve it. I am generally the last one off the practice field.

The final element of trust—constancy—exists when the performer knows that he or she can count on the coach, that the coach is at practice sessions with the team and stays until the end of the game even through a discouraging and dismal loss. The coach does not bow out and head for the locker room early just because the team is behind. Observation of team and individual performance is not possible if the coach is not at the game. Videotaping is a wonderful way of replaying performance, but it is not the same as being there. No sports coach worth his or her salt waits until after the game to review performance and give corrective feedback.

Mutual Respect

A good relationship requires mutual respect. The coach's job is to push players toward their peak performance. Players need to believe that the coach has something to offer and is focused on helping them improve. When the coach's motivation is to help the team members be their very best, players may not like what the coach asks them to do, but they respect it. "Lots of leaders want to be popular, but I've never cared about that. I want to be respected. Respect is different from popularity. You can't make it happen or demand it from people, although some leaders try that. The only way you can get respect is to earn it" (Shula and Blanchard, 1995, p. 50).

Players do not highly value being pushed to satisfy the coach's ego. A women's collegiate volleyball team provides a good example of this. The coach had recently graduated, and this was her first coaching job. She drove the team mercilessly because she wanted a championship team in her first year out of school. Her relentless pursuit of this goal in spite of the fact that the team just did not have the experience or ability necessary led to her complete ineffectiveness as a coach. By the end of the year, she did not have enough players left to take the court as a team. The players knew that she was not interested in helping them improve their performance for any reason other than her ego's needs.

Communication

Communication is the final requirement for a healthy relationship between a coach and performer. Readers can view issues and principles of communication discussed fully in Chapter Four for their applicability to coaching. Without the ability to articulate direction, vision, and goals and to give feedback, the coaching process simply does not work. Good communication skills are the vehicle through which the leader carries out the coaching process. Communication that is direct, honest, and predominantly positive generates a healthy coaching relationship. If the person being coached hears mostly negative feedback, the relationship begins to deteriorate.

Perhaps as important as the quality of the relationship between the coach and performer is the definition, or structure, of the relationship. Role definition and agreement are essential, especially in the workplace, where nebulous coaching relationships exist.

Establishing the specifics of the coaching role, what it entails, what areas it includes, and what approaches the coach will use adds clarity to an otherwise vague process. The coach and performer work out the coaching agreement together to ensure mutual understanding of the various roles. A structured coaching relationship elevates what is often a casual and sporadic process to a consistent, development-focused process.

Motivation

Understanding and applying the principles of motivation are inherent elements of the coaching role of an effective leader. Influencing others requires comprehension of the reasons people act in certain ways. *Motivation* is what causes a person to act in a particular manner. There are a multitude of theories related to motivation, and all have relevance for the leader seeking to better understand a follower's nature. These theories include need-fulfillment (Maslow's hierarchy of needs), Herzberg's two-factor theory (what satisfies does not necessarily motivate), expectancy theory (a person behaves in a certain way if he or she believes the effort will yield a reward), and equity theory (one determines expected outcomes by comparing one's work and rewards to others doing a similar job). Rather than reviewing these theories, which readers can find in almost any text on organizational behavior and development, this section briefly reviews some common misconceptions about motivation, the factors related to intrinsic motivation, and two major principles of motivation applicable in a coaching situation. The first is the principle of expecting the best, and the second is knowing the desired outcome and then reinforcing it by reward.

Misconceptions About Motivation

Anyone seeking to influence another person needs to be skilled at motivating. McGinnis (1985) describes several of the many common misconceptions about motivation and offers examples to refute them.

- *All motivation is intrinsic.* Perhaps the most common misconception is that no one can motivate another person and that all motivation comes from within. For years managers have heard: "You cannot motivate another person; all you can do is create an environment that is motivating." Although intrinsic motivation is very powerful, it is not the only source of motivation. Everyone remembers an instance in which the presence of someone else—an inspiring teacher, a dynamic and encouraging coach, or simply the presence of loved ones—led to increased performance, even performance beyond expectation. McGinnis (1985) cites several historical examples, such as Wellington reporting that when Napoleon was on the field, it was like fighting an additional forty thousand men. Winston Churchill's leadership breathed hope into a dispirited and frightened England during the last seven months of 1940 and changed the future of the modern world.

- *Some people just are not motivated.* Everyone is motivated, though it may be by and for different things. The employee who is usually late and takes an extra half hour to get rolling in the morning may be the first one out the door in the afternoon, full of enthusiasm! The fifteen-year-old who requires continual nagging to get out of bed on a school morning can get himself up and out of the house at 4 A.M. on Saturday for a fishing trip with friends. These two have plenty of motivation—it is just inspired by particular things. The challenge for the leader is to channel that already existing energy into endeavors good for the team or organization.

When first introduced to the idea of shared decision-making models for employees, whether in self-directed or self-managed work teams or governance structures, many managers and supervisors react with skepticism. From their years of observing employee behavior, these leaders simply cannot conceive of employees accepting more responsibility willingly, such as participating in peer review, self-scheduling, managing inventory and supplies, or jointly interviewing applicants for an open position in the department. Most employees in a bureaucracy learned long ago that getting involved beyond the minimum required in a day's work simply does not pay. But when they realize that they really can, and are allowed to, make decisions that directly affect their work life, their enthusiasm returns. Most people prefer having control over their lives.

- *Motivation is manipulation.* In its negative connotation, *manipulation* is when a person tries to persuade another to a certain course of action that is not to the individual's benefit but to the motivator's benefit. Genuine motivation is finding mutually beneficial goals that are good for both individuals and then forming a satisfying partnership to achieve these goals.

- *Motivational people are born, not made.* Contrary to this final misconception, anyone can become an effective motivator. It simply takes an understanding of the theories and basic principles. This is good news for leaders wanting to further develop their effectiveness.

Applying the principles of motivation increases the leader's ability to influence others. The following section offers a framework for understanding intrinsic motivation as well as identifying and explaining two primary principles of motivation.

Understanding Intrinsic Motivation

The intrinsic motivators are those elements within us that influence our behaviors. If motivation is what makes us do what we do, then intrinsic motivation consists of those internal factors that result in our taking a particular course of action. Although it sounds paradoxical, a good leader understands these and takes action to build on them, thus applying the added influence of external motivation.

Thomas (2000) offers a solid conceptual framework for understanding these intrinsic motivators and offers a compelling case for their contribution and importance in today's work world. "The new work role is more psychologically demanding in terms of its complexity and judgment, and requires a much deeper level of commitment. While economic rewards were pretty good for buying compliance, gaining commitment is a far different matter" (p. 5).

He clearly believes that external motivators such as money and benefits are no longer enough to compel workers to act. When intrinsic motivators are present, an individual is more likely to feel energized and vibrant in his or her work. The five intrinsic motivators are the presence of healthy relationships, a meaningful purpose, competence, choice, and seeing progress.

Recent work in the field of positive psychology has further substantiated much of the work on intrinsic motivators. Studies on happiness have found that there are three elements to happiness in life: pleasure, engagement, and meaning (Seligman, 2002). And to live the fullest life means that these three elements are present in all aspects of our lives: within ourselves, in our life with those we love, and in our work life.

Healthy Relationships

People are clearly more highly motivated to perform in a particular way if they have a positive, healthy relationship with others in the workplace. It is very unlikely that a person goes the extra step for someone he or she actively dislikes or does not respect. Because healthy working relationships were examined more fully in Chapter Two, this discussion will not do so. Suffice it to say, the establishment of positive relationships and a sense of connection to the people in our workplace leads to higher intrinsic motivation.

Meaningful Work

"People have a desire to be engaged in meaningful work—to be doing something they experience as worthwhile and fulfilling" (Thomas, 2000, p. 12). Many of us have work that is composed of tasks that serve a particular end or accomplish a specific purpose. When we are clear about what the purpose is, we can make intelligent decisions about the work. Rather than seeing work as a necessary evil, or something that costs us, we find work itself meaningful and rewarding.

A second-career nurse was being interviewed for a research project and was questioned about her experience of joy through her

work. Her current job was in the outpatient recovery area of a diagnostic center. In the course of the interview, she mentioned casu-
ally that after almost six years, she was now nearing the salary level
she had left behind to enter a nursing educational program. She
went on to say that she would never go back to manufacturing, even
if the money was better, because her work as a nurse allowed her to
see each and every person for whom she made a difference. In her
words, our world "can live without chrome bumpers for our cars,"
but it could not survive without someone to care for the sick and
injured (Manion, 2002a). The meaningfulness of her work far out-
weighed the financial considerations.

Because the very nature of health care encompasses some of the
most meaningful work known to humankind, the care of others who
are sick and at their most vulnerable, we might assume that health
care work is inherently meaningful and think that, as leaders, we
need take no specific action in this area. There are, however, several important ramifications. The first is that some individuals in
the organization may do such a narrow piece of work that they may
not see their connection to the contribution to the well-being of
patients—the volunteer who delivers patient mail, the maintenance
worker who puts a fresh coat of paint on the walls, or the house-
keeper who circulates and empties the trash. The leader can help
everyone see his or her contribution and the importance of the work.

Secondly, the leader, along with employees, must be continually
alert to events or situations that indicate the organization is not living up to its stated mission and values. When organizational decisions and behaviors contradict what employees believe is the
organization's mission, the resulting dissonance can severely affect
the person's sense of meaning. And finally, especially in today's
health care organizations, leaders must continually seek to reduce
the amount of work perceived as near meaningless that creeps into
the job. Few health care workers choose their field because they
wanted to spend half of their time documenting and recording what
they did. The impact of increased regulation in health care has

resulted in greater focus on paperwork and compliance with arbitrarily established rules—often at the cost of time spent in the delivery of actual service in the department. Add to this the amount of duplicative work and time employees spend cleaning up the problems of other departments, and you can see that we are quickly reaching the tipping point when health care workers begin to believe that the meaningless has overtaken the meaningful work in their day.

Competence

"You have a sense of competence on a task when you feel that you are performing your work activities well—when your performance of those activities is meeting or exceeding your own standards" (Thomas, 2000, p. 77). Most of us are more likely to enjoy work at which we are good. Seligman (2002) defines authentic happiness as knowing our signature strengths and crafting a life that uses these strengths in all aspects, personally and at work. In other words, we are more likely to be happy engaged in work that taps into our abilities and reflects our competence.

Csikszentmihalyi has done extensive research on the concept of flow (1990, 1997, 2003). He defines *flow* as an optimal experience that is the unintended side benefit of engaging in activities in which we are stretched to our limits by challenges that are worthwhile. It is both a sense of mastery and involvement or participation in an event. "Flow is the state in which people are so involved in an activity that nothing else seems to matter; the experience itself is so enjoyable that people will do it even at great cost, for the sheer sake of doing it" (1990, p. 4). Competence is an important part of this concept; the situation calls for a stretch on our part. If there is not enough challenge to our abilities, boredom or apathy is the result. And if the challenge exceeds our ability to master it, frustration is the result.

The ramifications of personal competence for health care leaders are far-reaching. First, this intrinsic motivator provides ample justification for the inclusion of this chapter as an important contribution to increasing the leader's interpersonal competency. The role of the leader as coach is to help followers increase their level of competence, whether technical or interpersonal. Providing opportunities, learning about resources, emphasizing growth, and ensuring an organizational philosophy of continual learning are all important.

Another ramification has to do with selecting the right person for the right work or helping an individual resculpt work that does not use his or her competencies or signature strengths. Buckingham and Coffman (1999, p. 148) say that "casting is everything": "If you want to turn talent into performance, you have to position each person so that you are paying her to do what she is naturally wired to do. You have to cast her in the right role." This message was reinforced by Jim Collins's research (2001, p. 41) studying why some organizations were able to make the leap from being good to exceptional performers: "The executives who ignited the transformations from good to great did not first figure out where to drive the bus and then get people to take it there. No, they *first* got the right people on the bus (and the wrong people off the bus) and *then* figured out where to drive it." Furthermore, when determining who the right people are, the greater emphasis is on character attributes rather than specific experience or education (Collins, 2001; Manion, 2004b). Having specific skills or knowledge is important, but exceptional leaders know that these are teachable, whereas character traits are more ingrained.

Crafting work that fits an individual is another aspect of the leader's role. Loehr and Schwartz (2003) have extensive experience in coaching both sports athletes and corporate athletes (their term for performers in the work world). They share example after example of individuals who came to them for coaching because they were exhausted and nearly depleted of energy. These people had lost a sense of connection and competence in their work. Sorting through what they are extremely good at is a key aspect of redefining the work so that it engages a person's full capabilities (Loehr and Schwartz, 2003; Seligman, 2002).

Another potential role of the leader is in creating work environments that are more likely to lead to optimal experience or flow on the part of employees. Flow is also engagement; in fact, when we are in flow, we are so engaged that we do not even notice time passing. A quick examination of most health care workplaces reveals multiple barriers to the experience of flow. Workers experience countless interruptions of work, whether through beepers and cell phones, overhead announcements, environmental noise, and e-mails—all of which interrupt or prevent flow.

An important payoff when employees work with a sense of their own competence is that they feel pride. When Byrne (2003, p. 66) interviewed Jon Katzenbach about his latest book, *Why Pride Matters More Than Money*, Katzenbach said, "It's more important for people to be proud of what they are doing every day than it is for them to be proud of reaching a major goal. That's why it's crucial to celebrate the 'steps' as much as the 'landings.' The best pride builders are masters at spotting and recognizing the small achievements that will instill pride in their people." This is not the same as acting prideful in the sense of arrogance but is the positive emotion of feeling proud of one's accomplishments.

Choice

We feel a sense of choice on a task or responsibility when we see that our views, ideas, and insights matter. Choice also has to do with felt ownership, when we feel personally responsible for the outcome of our behaviors or decisions. "Choice takes on extra importance when we are committed to a meaningful purpose. Then a sense of choice means being able to do what makes sense to you to accomplish the purpose" (Thomas, 2000, p. 65).

A leader in today's workplace may not have any control over the individual's initial choice to be there, that is, whether the person must work or not. However, it was clear in the discussion on organizational commitment that people must feel they have a choice before they can feel engaged and committed to their work. A freely made choice to work in this particular organization is instrumental in employee's feelings of commitment. Beyond this, however, leaders have a great deal of control over this intrinsic motivator.

Models of shared decision making, operationalizing empowerment, and delegation are common ways to increase employees' exercise of choice in their work. Giving people the authority to make decisions that are within their scope of responsibility and trusting them to do so are important leader behaviors. Creating a climate that discourages placing blame and finds positive responses to mistakes are further ways a leader encourages followers to make decisions and show initiative.

Progress

A sense of progress occurs when you feel like your activities have the impact that you intended, when you see that your work is achieving its purpose. Little is more discouraging to us than to feel that nothing changes as a result of our effort and hard work. When we see progress, it creates momentum and enthusiasm; and the energy to continue onward becomes available to us. An ancient Greek legend portrayed the torture of Sisyphus, who was doomed to push a large boulder up to the top of a hill, then stand aside and let it roll back to the bottom. Then his work began again, pushing the boulder to the top. Such repetitive work with no appreciable outcome is the ultimate torture of a being who inherently seeks meaningful work.

The research on what brings people joy in their work clearly indicates that seeing results and making progress is essential (de Man, 1929; Manion, 2002a; Manion, 2003). The ramifications for health care leaders are many: we need to analyze and remove barriers to progress within our systems. For too many years, we have tolerated the same problems in our systems. Implementing an effective process improvement approach is not just the latest consulting fad or organizational culture change; instead, it is crucial if employees and leaders alike are going to have the tools to make both incremental and substantial change in our systems. Employees and leaders must share the responsibility for true process improvement. Many of the processes that Chapter Six identified (problem solving, appreciative inquiry, polarity management) are approaches for dealing with these issues.

In addition to putting into place effective processes for dealing with issues and problems, organizations must develop measurement and accountability systems so that people can track their progress and see their results. Accountability systems are notoriously weak in health care organizations. For example, with the current emphasis and focus on the leader's responsibility in recruitment and retention, few health care managers have access to department-specific measures of vacancy and turnover rates or satisfaction measurements by patients, employees, and physicians. Yet their organizations are holding these managers accountable for outcomes in areas where measurements are inadequate or so outdated as to be useless.

A final ramification for leaders to consider here is how they recognize and reward progress. If leaders do not even recognize progress, they cannot acknowledge it. In the late 1990s a hospital in the Southeast was positioning itself to become part of a larger health care system. In order to appear as financially viable as possible, administration asked each segment of the current system to make a substantial contribution by reducing its operating expenses. In the organization's large home health agency, the managers were expected to reduce their expenses by $1.2 million over the next year. These exceptional leaders worked closely with their employees in order to achieve this result. Employees were instrumental in designing and implementing a workforce reduction that was well received. In nine months the agency reduced expenses by $1 million.

The system CEO and chief financial officer called the two managers to a meeting to report on their progress. For an hour the executives badgered, questioned, and basically harangued the two departmental leaders to determine how they would reduce the remaining $200,000 of expenses. The executives neither mentioned the progress the managers had achieved nor commended them for the exemplary way they had obtained the current results. You can imagine the level of interest and motivation these two leaders felt when they left the meeting for their remaining task. In fact, both moved on from the organization within six months.

Celebrating and recognizing progress is not as easy as it sounds. We have reservations about celebrating too early. However, people pay attention to what we emphasize. A very successful leader reported that creating fun things to do was her way of emphasizing what she felt was important. For example, when new employees in her department complete their orientation period, she takes them out to breakfast, and she takes their mentors or preceptors out to dinner (Manion, 2004b).

Motivation Principles

When the leader understands the principles of intrinsic motivation, he or she can choose behaviors that support these important principles. The leader must likewise understand external motivation. Two of its most important principles are expecting the best and knowing what you want so you can reward it.

Expect the Best

In coaching, attitude is everything. To put it simply, coaches who like people and who believe that people have the best of intentions often get the best performance. It is a well-documented fact that people live up to the expectations they and others have of them. Henry Ford said it best: "Whether you think you can or you think you can't, you're right!" If the coach expects the best from his or her performers, that is what the coach gets. Good coaches do not waste time looking for and exposing their performers' faults. Instead, they look for strengths and abilities that others have overlooked, and they find ways to encourage these special talents. If the coach is constantly on the watch for the person's worst side, performers become defensive and self-protective, and the door to an effective coaching relationship closes.

The coach can quickly turn a person or team into what he or she expects of them. Take, for example, the manager-coach in this situation: Jim, the department manager, has recently had his scope of responsibility expanded through the additional assignment of two new departments. Over the past several months, Jim has been grooming Susan, a long-term employee, to move into an assistant manager position in one of these departments. Although she has been gradually assuming more responsibility, Jim does not really believe that Susan is yet ready to effectively make decisions that he spent years learning to make. However, he feels he has no choice because of the circumstances in which he finds himself. Jim has a short vacation planned but is concerned about what might happen in his absence. Sure enough, on his return, he learns that Susan has made a poor decision with significant negative ramifications for the department.

Jim's reaction will greatly influence Susan's future behavior. On the one hand, Jim can say, exasperatedly (even if only to himself): "I should have known better than to take any time off. I didn't think she was ready, but I didn't have any choice." To further reinforce this reaction, every time Susan asks for more responsibility or for less micromanaging on his part, he reminds her of the fiasco the last time she was left alone. And when he is gone for a day or longer, he makes a point to call in and check up regularly to see what's going on. Or he asks a fellow department head to check a couple of times throughout the day just to be certain things are OK. What's the message to Susan? What happens the next time Susan needs to make a decision on her own? How does Susan feel about herself?

On the other hand, Jim's can react to the situation based on his belief that Susan can accept responsibility and make good decisions. His reaction might then be more like this: "Susan, this decision was a mistake. It isn't like you. Let's take a look at what was happening and how you can clear this up. We won't make a big deal out of this, but I want to help you figure out what you might do differently next time. We all learn from doing, and if you're not making any mistakes, you're probably not making any decisions. And I want you to make decisions, because I know you have good judgment and can make good choices."

The leader's belief about people influences how he or she approaches these coaching situations. And these beliefs create a self-fulfilling prophecy, which begins with an assumption that is not necessarily true. But by believing it is true, the leader acts as if it is and creates a cycle of behavior that results in the very behavior he or she initially expected or feared (Figure 7.1). This concept explains how the principle of "expect the best" works. Research has documented extensively the validity of this concept and has further discovered that people prefer others to behave as they expect them to (McGinnis, 1985; *Productivity and the Self-Fulfilling Prophecy*, 1997). If a coach has a belief about an individual and the individual does not behave in a manner to support this belief, the coach becomes uncomfortable. For example, if an individual succeeds

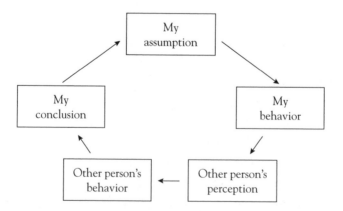

Figure 7.1. The Self-Fulfilling Prophecy

where a coach thought the individual would fail, this creates dissonant feelings in the coach.

The concept of the self-fulfilling prophecy is critical for workplace coaches because they have all kinds of expectations about the
people they work with, and some of these expectations are damaging. For example, executive leaders who believe that employees do
not want additional responsibility or involvement in decision making are less willing to share responsibility (Figure 7.2). A manager's
belief that employees without a professional education cannot manage themselves or are not as creative as employees with more education directly affects the degree of delegation that occurs. These
are common beliefs operating in today's workplace, and they limit
the potential of individuals' and teams' achievements. Effective
leaders continually seek to understand their own behavior to determine the presence of unrecognized negative assumptions.

Reward the Desired Behavior

The second major motivation principle involves rewarding the behavior we want to increase. To effectively influence others, the
coach must be crystal clear about the behavior he or she is seeking

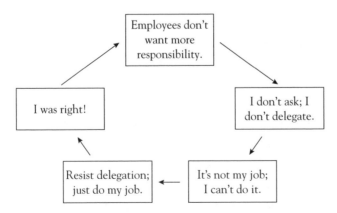

Figure 7.2. The Self-Fulfilling Prophecy in Action

and then reward that behavior. If the leader does not somehow reward or recognize the desired behavior, the follower will gradually stop behaving that way. Worse, if the leader rewards and reinforces contradictory behaviors, this results in poor outcomes, leaving leaders scratching their heads and wondering what happened.

The concept of reward is broader in scope than simply monetary rewards. Too often in the workplace, people assume that only money can be that reward. What is really needed is a variety of rewards. Money is certainly an important one, but it is often tied directly to the annual performance appraisal system. In too many organizations today, this system is more deflating than motivating. A large system in the Midwest implemented a new rating scheme for its annual performance appraisals. Department managers were told that roughly only one employee for every twenty should receive the highest rating. In one small department, the manager was directly advised that she could give only one of her employees this high rating.

The manager was in a dilemma because she had several exemplary performers, and she had to make a tough choice about who would receive the highest rating. One employee, Jane, had led a major housewide change initiative, coauthored an article for publication in a professional journal, and given a presentation at a national conference in addition to carrying her normal workload. Jane was devastated when her manager gave her a rating of average after a year of exceptional performance. Is it any wonder that employees disengage and remove themselves psychologically from their workplace? In this instance, the difference in money was negligible, but in terms of recognition for achievement, Jane felt this rating as a slap in the face. The organization unwittingly lost the commitment of one of its best members. Coens and Jenkins explore the inadvertent destruction of motivation created by contemporary performance appraisal systems in their book *Abolishing Performance Appraisals: Why They Backfire and What to Do Instead* (2000).

Good leaders use a variety of rewards, such as increased opportunity, going to lunch together, more individual time with the coach, increased flexibility in scheduling, visibility, praise, greater freedom, and even increased responsibility. These rewards are more likely to leave an individual with something to remember. Rewards are most effective when they come soon after the behavior or accomplishment the leader identifies and acknowledges. The leader must also offer the rewards sincerely.

Wells Fargo has developed innovative ways of rewarding people. At the year-end holidays, the organization gives employees a $50 bill. However, the stipulation is that each employee give his or her $50 to the coworker who had been the most helpful during the past year! What a wonderful way to reinforce cooperation and teamwork among coworkers. The company gave employees who received the most $50 bills a choice of another holiday gift. The list included items such as two pounds of Mrs. Field's cookies every month for a year, a two-hour body massage on April 15, a new puppy, or a menu item named in their honor in the Wells Fargo cafeteria. These gifts made a tremendous impact and were not soon forgotten.

A good coach is very careful to avoid rewarding behaviors contradictory to those desired. If, for instance, the leader always gives increased responsibilities to two or three employees because they are especially willing and competent, after a time these individuals may feel like they are pulling the weight for the whole team. If the leader considers raising issues and offering different viewpoints to be positive team behavior, then the leader should recognize and remark on that behavior rather than the compliant behavior of simply going along with everyone else. An executive in one organization was known for belittling and chastising people who offered opinions differing from his, yet he constantly verbalized the importance of speaking up and being honest.

A newspaper column some years ago gave a classic example of a punitive reward for good behavior. The nationally syndicated columnist Sandra Pesmen (1990, p. E21) received the following question: "I called my top commission salesman in another city last week and couldn't find him in the office or at any customer's offices. So I called his house at 1 P.M. and he answered the phone. When I asked what he was doing there, he answered that he'd filled his quota for the month, and if he worked any harder and made more sales, he'd just have to pay more to Uncle Sam. I'm furious but wonder what to do. He is a good rep, works well with our customers there and knows our line."

Pesmen's answer is insightful and representative of the mentality prevalent in some sectors of society: "Try and remember you're the boss. Cut his commission so he'll have to work harder to make the same personal profits. While he's doing that, he'll be increasing the company profits, which is the main goal. If he gets angry over that and quits, remember no one is indispensable" (1990, p. E21). So the bottom line here is that every time this salesman increases his sales, he will get less, not more. What is this company rewarding? And why would anyone in their right mind continue working hard for such a company?

Sometimes what we are rewarding is not quite so obvious. But it is a well-known fact that what we pay attention to and remark on is often what increases. "If you pay the most attention to your stragglers and ignore your stars, you can inadvertently alter the behaviors of your stars" (Buckingham and Coffman, 1999, p. 155). And when our best performers start slipping, it is a sign that we have been paying attention to the wrong people and the wrong behaviors.

These two basic concepts—building a healthy foundational relationship and applying the principles of motivation—increase the effectiveness of the leader involved in developing followers' skills and abilities. Some leaders understand these concepts inherently, but others may use this review as a reminder of their importance.

The Coaching Process

The most effective coaching process is based on a partnership relationship between coach and performer. The essence of the relationship is one of mutual benefit, an exchange of equal contribution between the two parties. Zemke (1996, p. 27) notes: "Managers who see themselves as coaches will also tend to see their employees as individuals of innate talent and worth. Managers who see themselves as coaches will strive to act as trusted advisers to help people develop those talents and use them in concert with others toward the achievement of a common and shared goal. Managers who see themselves as coaches tend not to think of their employees as vassals."

Indeed, active coach-leaders and coach-managers see themselves in partnership with performers. The coaching process includes these six steps:

1. Establish the purpose or goals.
2. Assess the performer's needs.
3. Reach agreement on expectations and parameters.
4. Teach or train for the desired skills.
5. Observe performance.
6. Give feedback.

Step One: Establish the Purpose or Goals

The first step of the process is to determine the purpose of the coaching. Why is the leader coaching the individual? Is there a performance gap issue? Does the individual need to improve performance simply to meet the expectations of the role or job? Is the leader trying to develop advanced skills in the performer? Is the leader evaluating the individual's strengths and capabilities to determine future promotion opportunities? Is the coaching part of a succession-planning strategy? The strongest goals are those that the coach and performer develop mutually. Goals that the leader develops for others are less likely to be embraced. The most common example of this occurs in disciplinary situations. Too often the manager creates a development plan and delivers it to the employee.

Without a specific goal in mind, coaching is less likely to be intentional and proactive, as we discussed previously. In some instances, the coaching plan is specific and concrete enough that the leader and follower write out and agree on the goals. For instance, the CEO coaches several members of the executive team so that they are able to attend and function effectively at key meetings with the board of trustees. A manager focuses on developing an employee to lead a department action committee for solving unique or difficult problems. Department leaders implementing a shared decision-making structure often use an explicit coaching plan for each group leader and each group.

In other instances, the purpose of the coaching is more general and nonspecific: it is simply a desire to intentionally focus on others' development needs. It is comparable to the reactive form of coaching we mentioned earlier. A situation arises spontaneously; and the coach naturally teaches, trains, or gives feedback on observation of the performance.

A coaching session usually involves discussing goals, which then become a frequent topic of conversation. They need to be brought out frequently and considered and reconsidered. Many of us have had the experience of approaching the time for our annual performance review and suddenly remembering that we have identified goals that have been sitting in a file cabinet somewhere for the past year. This kind of goal setting has little power to influence us positively.

The Gallup Organization has conducted extensive research with over eighty thousand managers who excelled at turning their employees' talent into performance (Buckingham and Coffman, 1999). They found that the manager who encourages employees' development takes the time to sit down and periodically find out what the employee is interested in and what his or her job aspirations are. Research conducted to determine what health care managers actually do day to day to create a workplace culture of engagement found that successful managers paid a great deal of attention to their employees' growth and development (Manion, 2004b).

Once the purpose or desired direction is clear, then the coach and performer determine the latter's precise needs by completing an assessment. Although assessment of the performer's needs is the second step of the coaching process, assessment is also inherent within each step. For instance, some level of assessment occurs before the partners determine the purpose or goal. Prior to teaching or training, assessment of appropriate interventions is necessary. And observing performance, the fifth step, entails assessing or appraising the results of the coaching to determine whether it was effective or not.

Step Two: Assess the Performer's Needs

The second step of an effective coaching process is assessment. It may be completed by the performer, the coach, or both. First, one identifies the desired skill or competency. In some instances, the performer becomes aware of a need for coaching in a specific area. It may be a new skill or job responsibility with which the individual has little or no experience, or circumstances may have changed significantly since the last time this individual accepted the responsibility. In other instances, the coach may have become aware of the need for coaching by observing a gap between actual performance and acceptable or exceptional completion of the responsibility.

However the need for coaching is identified, the focus of assessment includes appraising the performer's level of development or accomplishment of the task or responsibility. In their situational leadership model, Hersey and Blanchard (1993) have categorized four development levels that assist both coach and performer in assessing the individual or team and determining the most effective coaching intervention. They found that the most effective leader is the one who accurately assesses what the follower needs, based on the developmental level of the particular skill, and then provides what the follower is lacking.

Patricia Benner (1984) has conducted extensive research on how clinicians, specifically nurses, learn their clinical skills. She found that nurses progress through five stages of development as they learn their practice: novice, advanced beginner, competent, proficient, and expert. The practitioner is substantially different in each of these stages in several ways. First, as a novice, the individual relies on concrete, rigid principles; as skill acquisition occurs, the person begins to rely on actual experience. Consider, for example, when an individual is first learning a new skill such as playing racquetball. You learn exactly how to hold the racquet and to follow through with your swing. As you become more proficient, you no longer think about these details; instead, you shift your weight and handle the racquet based on what is going on in the game.

A second way we differ in these stages of development is in how we perceive the situation. A novice is often overwhelmed by all of the details in a given situation and often cannot act quickly enough. With years of experience, the person is able to quickly assess a situation, even as it unfolds, and determine what is the most important action to take first and what should follow. To return to the previous example, anyone who plays racquetball can remember the first time on a court and the feeling of panic and bombardment as the ball bounces from wall to ceiling to floor to ceiling again, often so quickly that it is difficult to follow. As you become skilled in the sport, you develop a sense for the ball and a focus on strategy.

The skill acquisition model dovetails nicely with a situational leadership model. Both respect the development of the individual and recognize the changing needs of the performer. The leader must consider the follower's skill and ability in a given situation in order to provide the appropriate leadership intervention. Two different people in the same situation may need entirely different coaching.

To return to the situational leadership model, each level is based on two aspects: the performer's competence and commitment. Competence refers to the performer's knowledge, skill, and experience. Commitment includes the performer's willingness to perform or interest in accepting the responsibility or task, the performer's confidence, and the level of the performer's motivation. The following sections describe the four development levels along with the coaching interventions to help the individual realize what he or she may need.

Development Level One: Novice

This is a new responsibility for the individual. The person may have had education and theory but no or very limited actual experience or practice with the skill or responsibility. Performers at this level are usually excited and enthusiastic about trying a new skill. Thus, the competence level is low, but commitment is high.

Coaching interventions include sharing any information that the performer needs. This includes telling the performer what to do and how, where, and when to do it. It can include making educational opportunities available to the individual, suggesting reading resources, or even recommending practice with a specialized coach. However it is accomplished, the coaching intervention is to provide the competence that the performer lacks. Commitment and enthusiasm are high, so the performer needs little encouragement.

Any information that the coach provides is very structured and detailed, with the coach closely controlling and monitoring the situation because the performer does not yet have well-established skills. In fact, too many explanations and examples can cause confusion because the performer needs only the basics at this stage.

Development Level Two: Advanced Beginner

This is a higher development level because the performer has had some experience using this skill or taking on this responsibility but is not yet accomplished. Perhaps the situation in which the task must be applied is new. Commitment is variable because after trying something and not having things proceed as well as expected, the performer may feel discouraged and frustrated to learn that the task is not as easy as he or she first believed. As a result, the performer lacks self-confidence and may even resist the idea of trying again.

At this level, the performer has some competence but low commitment. The coach's role is to furnish the additional technical competence the performer needs and plenty of enthusiasm and support. In addition to the how-tos of level one, the coach adds personal examples and perhaps discloses his or her own early difficulties in gaining the particular skill. The coach asks questions about the performer's experiences and previous successes and listens carefully to the answers. This provides an opportunity to redirect or reinforce behavior. Thus, the leader-coach provides what is missing: encouragement to bolster the performer's commitment and direction to support knowledge and skill.

Guided discussions are very appropriate at this stage because the performer may be making progress without realizing it and may simply need someone with an objective viewpoint to recognize that and point it out. When used with praise and positive reinforcement, this reinforcement can provide the encouragement the performer needs.

Development Level Three: Competent

At the competent level, the performer is experienced in applying the skill or has the competency required to assume the responsibility but has variable commitment. The individual may have high proficiency in this skill but in a completely different setting and may lack confidence in that ability because he or she does not recognize its transferability, or the people involved may be new to the performer. This performer is high on competence but variable on commitment.

At this level, the performer is competent, and any information or knowledge the coach provides is minimal, often limited to key parameters and expectations that apply. For example, the only structure the coach gives may be to share the final date by which the performer is to complete the task or identify key constraints, such as budget limitations or expected stakeholder involvement. The performer is fairly experienced with this responsibility and just needs a coach available to talk through ideas and possible solutions.

However, commitment is variable at this point. The performer has wavering confidence in his or her ability to achieve the desired outcomes. The current situation may be significantly different from any in his or her experience or simply more complex or difficult than usual. Whatever the case may be, at this point the coach provides much-needed encouragement and support through guided discussions, asking questions and listening carefully to answers, and reminding the performer of previous successes and lessons learned. With a highly competent performer, the focus is that little extra push of encouragement and confidence that a trusted coach can give. The coach remains available to the follower.

Development Level Four: Expert

This is the highest level of development that a performer achieves. Experience in the performance area is broad enough that the individual has not only the technical competency but a high level of judgment in applying the skills. Additionally, commitment is high. The performer is motivated, confident, and enthusiastic about the responsibility.

For the highly competent and committed performer, the coach really does not need to provide much of anything. There may be a need to provide the barest of structure—perhaps clarification of a time frame or key parameters and constraints. The coach and performer often negotiate these, as would be expected in an equal partnership.

Although recognition and rewards are always important, they are less important to the performer at this level of development. Much of the commitment and enthusiasm is generated from profound intrinsic motivation. As in development level one, the performer has plenty of zeal and is excited about the task to be accomplished.

Completing the Assessment

Ways in which to assess a performer's development level include observing actual performance, self-reporting by the performer, and gathering information coming from third-party sources. Yet another source of information may be knowledge of the logical process. For example, if an individual has performed well as a leader of a department, the next step in his or her development might include leadership opportunities of cross-department or cross-divisional projects or problem-solving groups. If an executive leader has performed well and mastered his or her responsibilities within the organization, the next step may be opportunities that are systemwide.

Accurate assessment is crucial because the individual's development level determines the coaching intervention the situation requires. If the assessment is inaccurate, the resulting intervention may range from ineffective to downright harmful. For instance, if the performer is at development level one and is low on competence, the coach's role is to provide access to needed knowledge and information. If the coach erroneously assessed the individual at development level three with a high level of skill and the coach determines that the performer needs only encouragement and support, the coach falls short. The performer then becomes frustrated and demoralized by not performing at the expected level.

A good example of this was observed in an organization undergoing massive change. A special project team of employees was identified and assigned to the project for a two-year period. The team's purpose was to lead the organization's major change initiatives. Tom was appointed team leader. Having received his master's degree in hospital administration, Tom had recently completed his administrative residency at the hospital. A tall, imposing figure who dressed for corporate success, Tom exuded confidence and capability without being arrogant. He was a relatively young man, however, having completed his master's work immediately following his undergraduate program; and he had no hands-on management experience.

Leaders erroneously believed that Tom was at development level three in terms of managing the team because he had significant leadership experience, and he certainly looked the part. Unfortunately, people overevaluated this promising young man repeatedly. Not only did he not receive the specific, basic managerial skill development and direction he needed, but when he did not meet people's unrealistic expectations, he had to face their extreme disappointment and negative reactions. Tom was in a no-win position.

The same can happen with children. In one family, both the father and mother were very tall. Their young son grew rapidly, and at six years, he towered over all of his friends, his appearance easily that of a child twice his age. The mother reported being embarrassed and concerned by the judgmental comments and behaviors of other people who assumed that this six-year-old behavior was coming from a twelve-year-old! Her son's behavior was very appropriate for his age but unacceptable to others who had assessed him based on a cursory glance and had come to very inaccurate conclusions.

Inaccuracies in assessment also occur in the opposite direction. When the individual or team has a higher level of competency than the leader believes and the leader provides more detail and direction than the performer needs, the performer is irritated and concludes that the leader is micromanaging or afraid to relinquish control. When teams or individuals are at developmental level three or four, they are highly competent. If the leader closely monitors and supervises their work (appropriate behavior for levels one and two), resentment and anger often result.

Step Three: Reach Agreement on Expectations and Parameters

Once the partners have clearly established the goals and direction and completed an appraisal of the performer's needs, the next step is to identify and agree on expectations and applicable parameters. Clarifying the operant expectations helps prevent misunderstandings. Expectations between coach and performer may include the role of each person as well as the most helpful desired approaches and behaviors. The coach must clearly identify parameters, and the performer must understand them. This section examines each of these issues with examples to illustrate their relevance within a coaching situation.

Expectations: Roles and Responsibilities

Early discussions about the roles and responsibilities of each party in a coaching relationship are essential. When the coaching relationship is a legal agreement between parties, the parties make the roles particularly clear. The conductor of a symphony orchestra regularly practices with the musicians and is responsible for procuring the best possible performance from them. The athletic coach is employed for the same reason: to develop individual team members to work as a team that will achieve peak performance. But relationships in the workplace are less clearly defined. Some coaches are very effective in developing performers yet are not in management positions. And many managers today see their coaching role as additional to their other responsibilities, something they do haphazardly and only when they have time, if at all.

Thus, an increasingly greater number of performers in today's workplace are unclear about the coaching role and may actually resent someone else observing their performance. In fact, their experience with the manager as a coach is limited to the annual performance appraisal or the less frequent (hopefully) disciplinary action. And leaders often handle these processes unsatisfactorily.

A conversation about the respective roles and responsibilities of each party formalizes the relationship and moves it from incidental and accidental to intentional. This objective consideration of who does what reduces the likelihood of strong emotions hampering the process. A coach's role is to facilitate or support the performers' development of skills by observing their performance and providing honest, direct feedback; by giving advice and instruction; and by encouraging discovery through guided discussions and hands-on experiences. The performer's role is to practice, perform, and use the coach's feedback, guidance, and instruction to further improve performance.

Expectations: Desired Approaches and Behaviors

Expectations concerning desired approaches and behaviors include such elements as the type of coaching required and the ways in which the coach will observe performance or deliver feedback. In discussions, coach and performer can clarify expectations and needs related to specific behavior. This actually forms an operating agreement. For example, the coach gives the individual immediate feedback after observing performance. But what qualifies as immediate feedback—within a few minutes, a few hours, or several days? Is it important that the coach deliver the feedback privately? Are voice-mail and e-mail messages acceptable? Is feedback kept confidential? Will there be time to discuss the feedback and ask questions? What does the coach expect of the performer who is receiving feedback? Is the performer to incorporate the suggestions and corrections in the next performance? Is the performer to receive the feedback with an open mind and a willingness to try alternatives?

Expectations and agreement on coaching interventions are determined by the performer's needs and are an important point to discuss. Ideally, in a healthy coach-performer relationship, the parties discuss the results of any assessment and reach an agreement on specific coaching interventions that the coach will provide. Even the most highly skilled performer has a need, at times, for direction and instruction. If the current situation is new to the performer, ways to increase knowledge and competence are the focus of the coaching. No matter how capable a performer, today's workplace is continually presenting new challenges for which performers need to develop competency. A performer may gain such competency if the performer's present and previous experiences are very similar, but the need for direct instruction and advice are paramount in the rapidly changing health care environment today.

One situation in a western health care system is a classic example. Ellen, the system's CEO, knew that as the system expanded to integrate a freestanding rehabilitation facility, a large home health facility, and a physician practice clinic, she could prepare for her own role changes by selecting a chief operating officer whose focus would be primarily on hospital operations. The final candidate came from her executive staff. Don, a young man, had the necessary educational qualifications and demonstrated leadership abilities. His current responsibilities included the marketing function and physician relations in the organization. When Ellen made the appointment, she was well aware that his downside was lack of experience and knowledge of hospital operations. In making her decision, she

was clear about her coaching role with Don. He would need direc-
tive interventions and learning opportunities to assist him in developing these competencies.

When the coach will provide competence and skill, there can
be emotional elements—both negative and positive—to consider.
Don was excited and pleased about his promotion because of Ellen's
trust and confidence in his abilities. If Ellen and Don had not talked
about his learning needs and the appropriate coaching interventions, he might have felt uncomfortable with the high level of
direction that Ellen would provide. There is added pressure from
Don's wanting to perform well after receiving such a big promotion.
This was a time of increased vulnerability for Don, with others
watching to judge the appropriateness of the promotion. He felt a
strong need to perform capably and competently to show himself
worthy of Ellen's trust.

In any department, implementing an employee team or council
structure provides a multitude of examples illustrating the importance of discussing appropriate coaching interventions. When organizations implement shared decision making models, they often
underestimate the coaching needs of the new groups. Many managers and leaders make erroneous assumptions about the group's
level of development. If individual department employees were at
a high development level, one may wrongly assume that their
group's development level is also high. But although group members' skills and competencies certainly influence the group's ability,
the two are not the same. Cherniss and Goleman (2001) clearly
report this when talking about a group's emotional intelligence. The
presence of a few emotionally intelligent members does not make
the team emotionally intelligent.

These false assumptions are often reinforced by highly skilled,
professional, and capable team members who believe that their individual high performance automatically translates to group high performance. In early stages of group development, the group needs a
manager-leader who provides the competence that the collective

entity lacks: how to work as a team or an effective group. Yet unless the group and manager-leader discuss the role of the coach and his or her assessment, the group or team may feel that the manager is giving a mixed message: "You said we're going to be responsible for making the decisions, so why are you telling us what to do?" Everyone involved feels they have failed and been failed because the situation does not meet their expectations.

Sometimes these issues and the need to talk through and agree on expectations become clear during the process of working together. In the beginning the parties assume many of these behaviors, but the danger of not talking through expectations is that they are much more difficult to discuss once either party has violated them. The performer may have assumed that the coach would give negative or corrective feedback privately, only to discover that the coach is giving critical feedback in the middle of an employee meeting. It is better to have a discussion prior to the occurrence of problems to prevent negative emotional reactions that can make effective resolution more difficult.

Relevant Parameters

The coach identifies any constraints, limitations, deadlines, or other parameters for the performer. If the coach does not think these through and share them with the performer, this can adversely affect outcomes; and the performer's enthusiasm and commitment may spiral downward, making the performer feel as though he or she has failed. Some individuals perform acceptably without this clarification, but this is not a chance worth taking—unless, of course, the coach is trying to assess the performer's ability to sort out and determine these important boundaries (which in itself can be a useful skill).

In a major system on the eastern seaboard growing in both size and scope, the CEO began delegating more and more responsibility to the chief operating officer (COO). The COO took on a major project: a patient safety initiative for the acute-care hospital facility.

This initiative was the CEO's favorite and important project. Instead of the CEO actively coaching the COO, it was a sink-or-swim affair. The CEO covered key constraints and expectations only loosely or assumed that the COO understood them. The COO misread and reversed the importance of many of these key parameters and forced the project through in an unrealistic time frame without adequate resources. The resulting negative impact on physician and customer satisfaction—the parameters most important to the CEO and board of trustees—eventually cost the COO his job. Clarifying expectations and parameters at the beginning of the coaching process can avoid this kind of demoralizing result.

In another organization the chief nurse executive was asked to become executive sponsor for a massive process improvement project that included the implementation of the universal room concept (where a patient is admitted to a bed and remains in that room and department for the duration of his or her hospitalization with needed services and level of care brought to the patient rather than the patient being transferred to other departments). This was her most important large-scope project since she had assumed her role eighteen months before. Her coach told her that the most critical parameter was that the project have no negative impact on physician or employee satisfaction ratings during its implementation. Based on everything she knew about change and the organization's relationship with physicians, this was an unrealistic expectation. As she accepted the responsibility, this expectation was a major discussion point. She negotiated much more realistic expectations, including an acceptable depth of decline in physician satisfaction scores over a reasonable length of time due to the change.

In another instance, a CEO told a chief nurse executive that he and his department would attain Magnet designation (which is conferred upon hospitals with exemplary nursing practice) for the hospital within twelve months. The nurse executive carefully investigated and developed a plan and a list of necessary resources and returned to the CEO to say, "This is what it will take to accomplish this goal within this time frame." As a result, not only did the organization establish a more realistic time frame, but it allocated important supports and resources.

The specificity of parameters is related to the performer's development level. At level one, the performer needs more detailed information. As the performer gains in experience and skill level, parameters become fewer or less concrete. For instance, when the performer is at level three, the structure that the coach gives may be only a time deadline or budget constraint.

An employee decision-making team leading the department redecoration process in one hospital decided to purchase beautiful color-coordinated linens for the patient rooms—bedspreads, curtains, draperies, and bed linens. To everyone's dismay, they discovered that the organization's laundry equipment could not process the particular fabric blend they had chosen. So these wonderful decorator linens sat in a warehouse, unused. It became an organizational example of why empowerment does not work and why employees cannot make decisions such as these. Granted, someone on the team could have suggested getting input from the experts in linen services, but a thorough coach would have identified the important parameter that the organization's laundry equipment must be able to process the linens! Or the coach might have identified a parameter that the team involve an expert from the linen service department before making a final decision.

A major difficulty is that leaders frequently imply rather than state expectations and parameters and assume that those involved understand and agree on the important expectations. This increases the likelihood that one or the other party involved in the coaching agreement fails to meet the other's unstated expectations. No matter how highly intuitive the participating individuals, they probably cannot read someone else's mind! The various people involved must clearly articulate and agree on expectations, needs, and parameters.

Step Four: Teach or Train for the Desired Skills

The fourth step of the coaching process is to teach or train for desired skills. Teaching others is also a specific manner in which a coach develops others and as such is discussed more fully under its own heading in this chapter. But because it is also a step in the coaching process, it is discussed here briefly.

Once the coach and performer have determined the purpose of coaching and completed the assessment, it becomes clear what specific skill development is necessary, either individual competencies or group and team skills. A good coach requires both individual and team practice. Individual practice focuses on increasing the proficiency of the individual's performance. Group or team practice is preparation aimed at the collective functioning of the group and its ability to orchestrate individual talents among them in order to deliver a fine performance.

The coach determines what to teach and when and how best to teach it. The *what* encompasses both technical or professional and supportive skills. Technical or professional skills pertain to the elements of an individual's job or work, such as completing a budget analysis or preparation, doing a counseling session with an employee, or preparing a collaborative strategic plan. Supportive skills are more general in nature, such as the emotional intelligence competencies of displaying empathy, communication, and coaching skills.

Selecting a teaching approach is paramount. Too often coaches use the methods of didactic classroom-style teaching and formal academic programs. Although these are valuable, coaches often overlook other possibilities. Tape recording and videotaping are powerful methods of instruction that can provide immediate, objective feedback on performance. Videotaping a meeting and replaying it to learn from participants' performances provide powerful lessons in group process. In one hospital's information services department, the clinical support team decided to tape record conversations with customers (with the customers' permission) to evaluate the team's effectiveness in handling complaints and support on the help line.

In considering how to teach or train a performer, an effective coach capitalizes on every teachable moment. It is as much an attitude as a technique. Using the day-to-day environment and continually seeking opportunities to demonstrate a point or teach a technique drives home the expectation that learning is an integral part of the workplace, not just something that happens in a classroom. The coach plans department and team meetings to include some teaching at each meeting. And teaching is not limited to what the coach provides. Exemplary performers also teach others, both formally and informally; and employees are therefore expected to coach and teach one another.

When to teach is more of an issue with regard to training in a formal learning setting such as a classroom. The most effective teaching and training are done at the time the skill or learning is needed, when the learner can apply it immediately and anchor it as a change in his or her behavior. However, most situations are not ideal; and the issue of when to provide training is fraught with difficulty. Training sessions and teaching most often occur prior to when they are actually needed or too long after the fact. This reduces the usefulness and adversely affects learning.

Step Five: Observe Performance

An active, involved coach spends a great deal of time simply watching people perform. If the coach dispenses with this necessary step of the process, the coach has no way of determining the success or effectiveness of the first four steps. Performers need to feel comfortable being observed. If the coach and performer have talked about the coach's role, the performer will receive the need for direct observation as a gift rather than interpreting it as micromanagement. The performer should see this as an opportunity to have an objective party provide feedback that will either reinforce good performance or correct faulty technique.

Direct observation is the best and preferred method for a coach to evaluate performance. Nevertheless, third-party reporting or self-reporting are acceptable. Third-party reporting may be negatively associated with tattling, which is unfortunate. This association has developed because many people are uncomfortable sharing criticisms or negative comments directly with the person they have observed and will instead share these observations with others. To avoid this negative connotation, keep sharing of third-party reports to positive observations. Everyone enjoys and appreciates hearing positive comments about his or her performance and values the third party who takes time to give positive feedback to the coach. The coach who receives negative third-party reports can use the information as an indication that he or she needs to do the observing and evaluating.

In the self-reporting process, the coach and performer talk through how a scenario played out, what the performer tried, what was effective, and what did not work. Asking questions that will draw out information in a comfortable, nonthreatening manner is important for this approach to work.

Another way the coach can evaluate performance is by evaluating actual outcomes against intended outcomes. Did the performer meet expectations? Were the outcomes acceptable or outstanding?

An advantage of observing performance directly is that the coach can evaluate the performer's ability. How long did it take the individual to learn the skill? What kind of teaching or training seemed to be most effective for this person? Did the performer demonstrate good judgment in asking for assistance during complex, difficult situations, or did he or she prefer to go it alone? Was the performer able to pace him- or herself appropriately? What work-load level can this performer handle? Does this individual feel comfortable negotiating modifications of workload? By observing performance, the coach learns a tremendous amount about the performer and becomes a more effective coach for this individual.

Step Six: Give Feedback

This step closes the loop and finalizes the entire process. Without providing feedback, the coach negates the whole process, leaving the performer with no way of determining the success or effectiveness of the first five steps. Having no feedback would be like playing a baseball game without innings or a scoreboard. A score of two to one in the bottom of the first inning is quite different from a score of two to one in the ninth inning, when the game is almost over and the chances for catching up are almost gone. In the same way that the score of a baseball game lets the team members know how they are doing, feedback lets performers know how they are doing.

The coach is, admittedly, only one source of feedback for good performers who are continual learners. They seek feedback from a variety of sources and are always evaluating their own performance. However, none of this other feedback can equal the value of honest, direct feedback from a trusted coach whose primary interest is in helping the performer to improve.

We give feedback through body language, through our reaction to situations, and even simply in what we give our attention to. In one organization a planning team made up of managers and executives was responsible for designing and making leadership development programs available. This team was responsible for everything: designing the content, engaging and preparing presenters, sending out invitations, and creating a positive learning ambience in the room on the day of the program. On this given day, they had worked especially hard to create a seasonal theme in decorating the room. Each table had beautiful fall centerpieces with special treats for the participants. Team members had made great efforts to create just the right atmosphere. The CEO walked in the room, took one look at the tables, and asked where the water pitchers were! His focus was on the item missing rather than all that the team had done. The entire team felt let down.

The same kind of feedback is given in a department when the leader arrives at work in the morning and rather than seeing all that the night employees surmounted and the challenges they overcame instead focuses with a critical eye on work that they did not complete. Attempting to get to the bottom of the problem with third-degree questioning, the leader gives clear feedback: the night crew failed. Leaders must be continuously aware of the feedback their behavior is giving to followers—whether purposeful or inadvertent.

This coaching discussion defines *feedback* more narrowly as giving information in the present about past behavior, in an effort to influence future behavior (Seashore, Seashore, and Weinberg, 1999). It is useful for leaders who want to influence the follower's behavior. "Feedback in the workplace is fundamental for helping those who wish to improve their performance, reach an objective, or avoid unpleasant reactions to their efforts" (p. 7).

To be effective, the feedback needs to be accurate. Expert coaches study the people they coach; they know them and look for strengths that others have overlooked. When small successes occur, they know how to transform them into larger successes (Buckingham and Coffman, 1999). The exemplary coach uses positive feedback, praise, and compliments, as well as redirection when necessary.

Positive Feedback and Praise

Nearly everyone wants to be appreciated and recognized for his or her performance. In fact, Smith (2003) says that the top motivator for employees is full appreciation for work well done, which managers express directly, either personally or publicly. In fact, Kouzes and Posner (2003) found that 98 percent of employees said they performed better when they received encouragement.

However, most positive feedback is general rather than intentionally specific about the behavior that it means to reinforce. Effective praise will reinforce that specific behavior. It is the difference between saying, "Thanks, you did a great job" and "Thanks, your persistence in getting the team to explore their differences has resulted in achieving consensus on this decision."

Tarkenton and Tuleja (1986) say that positive reinforcement for both normal behavior and exceptional performance is critical. They point out that people do a good job about four times as frequently as they do inadequate work. It makes sense, then, for anyone wanting improved results to recognize that performers do a good job at least 80 percent of the time. They say that negative feedback should be given in the same proportion. So an individual should receive praise at least four times as often as criticism. But almost the opposite is true, according to these authors: 80 percent of the typical feedback is based on the 20 percent that is poor performance.

Recent research in the field of positive psychology bears this out, finding that there is indeed a numerical ratio in the relationship of positive and negative feedback (Fredrickson, 2004). People need to hear good things about four to five times to every negative comment or experience in order to overcome the demoralizing effects of the negative comment.

Exemplary coaches are always seeking opportunities to give feedback; and in order to give praise, the coach must observe and catch the performer doing something right. Blanchard and Johnson (1981) are strong proponents of this philosophy. McGinnis (1985) offers several guidelines for giving praise:

- Hand out commendations in public.

- Use every success as an excuse for celebration.

- Use some gesture to give weight to the commendation.

- Put compliments in writing.

- Be very specific in praise.

McGinnis (1985) thinks that one problem with praise is that it can be overdone. If a person has established good, consistent performance and continues to be praised for the same thing, the praise soon becomes meaningless. The coach needs to find new behaviors to praise. A second challenge is that, if the coach has accomplished the first five steps of the coaching process and the performer shows signs of positive change, the coach must reinforce this new or changed behavior. It is terribly demoralizing to go to a great deal of effort to improve a skill or change a behavior and then realize that the coach doesn't even notice.

This last principle can be tricky when the behavior is in the right direction but the outcomes are not acceptable. One manager-coach was strongly urging a team to begin to take responsibility for solving problems and making decisions on team members' own initiative. The first decision they made was poor, mostly because it was limited in scope. The team had not considered the impact of their decision on other departments in the organization. The manager praised the fact that the team made a decision but then coached them through an evaluation of the outcome to help them see what key factors they had missed.

Negative Feedback

Giving negative feedback is often more difficult for coaches. "When you don't deliver critical feedback, you declare your indifference" (Clarke-Epstein, 2002, p. 79). Leaders who are reluctant to give a follower corrective feedback should ask themselves these questions:

> If I were the person in this situation, would I want to be told?
>
> With feedback, can the person change what's happening?
>
> Would the feedback be embarrassing for me to say or embarrassing for the other person to hear?

If the answer to the last question is yes, spend time carefully crafting the message.

Athletic coaches often use what is called a scolding coaching. This seems to work when the performer tries a skill or attempts a technique that does not work. The observant coach immediately redirects the individual by giving feedback known as scold instruction. The coach would say something like "Don't do it that way; do it this way."

Sometimes the performer needs a redirection or correction that is more negative. Blanchard and Johnson (1981) advocate giving one-minute reprimands, in which the redirection occurs quickly and honestly. Keep in mind the following steps in giving a redirection:

Do it immediately in order to correct the behavior as soon after it occurs as possible.

Confirm the facts with the individual before going further to ensure the information is accurate.

Be very specific and direct in saying what is wrong, focusing criticism on behavior rather than the person.

Show honest feelings so that the individual knows you are frustrated, angry, or disappointed.

A coach who is afraid to correct the performer's mistakes cannot be effective. When asked how he felt about negative feedback, one employee said, "I feel good when the feedback is positive, but I can change my behavior and improve my performance when it is negative. Hearing negative feedback may not be pleasant, but the results are more satisfying to me because it helps me more in the long run."

Coaching, then, is the primary means through which a leader can develop others. Intentional, proactive coaching involves performers using a specific process, including establishing the purpose, assessing, agreeing on expectations and parameters, teaching and training, observing performance, and giving feedback.

Developing Others Through Providing Opportunities

What may be one of the most powerful methods of developing others is also one of the simplest: providing opportunities. An exemplary leader continually seeks opportunities to stretch and challenge followers, reveling in others' accomplishments.

The extent to which a leader makes new opportunities available to followers demonstrates the importance the leader places on the development of new proficiencies. Furthermore, it delivers a high-impact message of trust and confidence in the follower's ability to perform well in a particular situation. Providing opportunities means seeking these occasions, presenting them to followers with enthusiasm and encouragement, removing barriers or obstacles, getting out of the way of the developing performer, and celebrating achievements.

This strategy was one that health care managers who had successfully created a workplace culture of engagement frequently identified. "I constantly seek opportunities for them." "Each employee has particular strengths and I seek to recognize those, asking them, what would they like to develop? What kinds of experiences would be beneficial to help prepare for the role they're pursuing?" (Manion, 2004b, p. 34).

Many high-performing leaders could undoubtedly look back over their own career paths and identify times when someone tapped them on the shoulder and asked them to take on a responsibility or task that they had not heretofore considered. Looking for ways to share the responsibility of leadership is one source of opportunities for followers. Is there a way to delegate some of the leader's responsibility? Exemplary followers continually seek challenge. However, their path is smoother and faster if an influential leader facilitates it by working on their behalf.

Removing barriers or obstacles for the follower is an important leadership responsibility, discussed briefly in Chapter Five. In the context of follower development, it might mean introducing the follower to the right person or simply speaking highly of the follower to other leaders in the organization. Recommending a follower to serve as the chair of an influential task force or committee, positioning the individual to receive appointments to boards or groups within the community or state—even promotions outside of the current position—are all ways a leader can remove barriers and champion followers. Many established and highly visible leaders receive more opportunities for service than they could possibly handle. Sharing some of these opportunities with followers is a way of supporting a follower's development.

If the leader is also the performer's manager, removing obstacles may mean something as rudimentary as providing time within the normal work week for the follower to engage in these other activities. Helping arrange for employee coverage, if necessary, and providing time away from the department to assume these new responsibilities is a way of saying to the follower: "I am serious about your development needs. They are important to me as well as to the organization."

In some instances, simply providing the opportunity is adequate; but most leaders also become involved in coaching the follower to help develop the individual's skills. If the leader is not able to provide what the follower needs, a referral or recommendation to another available coach may be effective.

A good leader is delighted, rather than threatened, when a follower's skill level surpasses the leader's own. The leader should treat achievement of outcomes and improvement of the performer's skills as occasions for celebration.

Teaching Others

Outstanding leaders are outstanding teachers. Noel Tichy addresses this concept clearly in his recent work with Nancy Cardwell, *The Cycle of Leadership: How Great Leaders Teach Their Companies to Win* (2002). They believe that institutions throughout society must have the capacity to develop leaders at all levels. Tichy and Cardwell call these teaching organizations with virtuous teaching cycles "dynamic, interactive processes in which everyone teaches, everyone learns and everyone gets smarter, every day" (p. xxiv). Regardless of their hierarchical position in the organization, leaders continually learn from each other and from followers.

In addition to holding a philosophy of continual learning, exemplary leaders also understand the principles of adult learning and are highly skilled in their application. Their teaching is intentional, and they engage in both spontaneous and deliberate teaching, obviously delighting in a follower's learning something new as well as their own learning. Such a leader lives by the old adage: give a man a fish and he eats for a day; teach a man to fish and he eats for a lifetime.

Here we review the principles of adult learning that effective leaders use to reinforce their application. Some people hear the word *teaching* and think of the familiar, formal academic model. But teaching is so much more than the traditional example of a teacher standing in front of a group and dispensing knowledge. The teaching-learning cycles that Tichy and Cardwell (2002) discuss occur continuously and simultaneously in the best learning organizations.

Most leaders today have been socialized and molded by an academic setting very different from what their children are experiencing. After years in an educational system with a relatively traditional approach, most adults expect to listen during the learning process while the experts teach them, disseminating information and giving advice. Ironically, it is not until the role of the educator shifts from transmitter of information to facilitator and resource person for self-directed inquiry that the learner will be able to meet his or her needs.

Principles of adult learning conjure images of participants in a learning situation who are actively participating. This means an active exchange of ideas, questioning, and perhaps hands-on practice. Active participation, however, does not necessarily mean that a person is continually interacting and talking. Participation can be as simple as thoughtful, private inquiry in reaction to something the teacher has asked or presented. In fact, there is growing appreciation of the power of reflective practice as a highly effective learning tool (Freshwater, 2004; Johns, 2004).

Taking generic principles or ideas that the teacher has presented and applying them to one's own situation is also active participation. In some instances, a teacher's example may create a vivid picture in a learner's mind that helps anchor the learning. So activity does not necessarily mean flashy exercises and dynamic situations that need a skilled facilitator for guidance.

Malcolm Knowles (1970) was one of the earliest educators in this country to distinguish between methods used for teaching children in a formal academic approach and those used for teaching self-directed learners such as adults. He described adult learning as differing from childlike learning in at least four main respects. First, the orientation to learning differs. Learning for children in school is often subject centered rather than problem oriented. The chief difference is in time perspectives. A child's perspective of formal education is one of postponed application, whereas an adult usually wants to apply his or her learning immediately. Compare a child's interest in a geography lesson about a country far away to the adult who is planning a vacation to that same country in the next four months. This issue of timing is critical. How many young people drop out of school because they do not see their learning experience as applicable and useful in their lives?

Change in a learner's self-concept is the second way that children's learning differs from adult learning. An assumption of self-directed learning is that as a person grows and matures, his or her self-concept moves from one of dependency to one of increasing self-confidence. Children are dependent on others in their earliest years, but as they grow and mature, they expect to participate more actively in decisions affecting learning. In fact, Knowles (1970) suggests that when adults find themselves in a situation in which they are not allowed to be self-directed, they experience tension between the given situation and their self-concept, resulting in resentment and resistance. They may think, *Why is this person telling me what to do? Does he or she think I don't know?*

The third area differentiating the two types of learning is the role of experience in learning. The assumption is that as an individual matures and accumulates experiences, these serve as resources for learning and an ever-enlarging base to which to relate new learning. Teachers convey their respect for students by making use of students' past experiences as a resource for learning. The learner's readiness to learn is the last point of difference that Knowles (1970) identified. As individuals mature, their readiness to learn is more the product of what they need to know, because of a change in their environment or life situation, than what others believe they ought to know.

Knowles's observations (1970) are powerful for those seeking to improve their teaching skills. In the same way that individuals are at varying levels of development related to the skill they are trying to learn, each is also at varying levels of development in learning. In other words, learning is a skill that one needs to develop. If we apply the assessment model for coaching provided earlier in the chapter, the different levels of learning might look like this:

- *Development level one.* This level of learning could be likened to the learning of a young child. Enthusiasm and commitment abound. The learner lacks competence and knowledge, so the teacher provides structure by deciding the appropriate curriculum and learning experiences required. The teacher provides required information and knowledge, guides the learning process, and evaluates outcomes.

- *Development level two.* At this level, the learner has some experience but variable commitment. Perhaps early attempts revealed that learning is not as easy as it seemed. This learner requires both strong direction and lots of support and encouragement. The instructor provides this direction, determining what to teach and how to teach it. At this point, most teachers remain actively present and involved during learning situations, giving feedback and attention as well as praise and encouragement.

- *Development level three.* The learner at this stage has fairly wide experience with learning but perhaps lacks self-confidence in the subject area. The learner needs minimal structure from the teacher, requiring mostly encouragement and support. The teacher uses guided discussions and practice or live sessions to facilitate learning.

- *Development level four.* This level represents the epitome of the self-directed learner. The learner is responsible for defining his or her own educational needs, necessary resources, and appropriate time schedules. The learner also undertakes evaluation of the learning process. At this level, the learner works in partnership with the teacher to appropriately define the learning outcomes expected and agree on an approach to learning. The self-directed learner has the ability to maturely evaluate educational materials and opportunities and effectively manages his or her own time.

Leaders in the workplace are working with followers who are typically at levels three and four. These learners are comfortable with learning and at level three may just need more coaching. These learners are the most likely to fall back into the more traditional modes of learning, such as didactic classroom presentations. Most leaders are blessed with at least some followers who are self-directed learners. These learners are open, curious, organized, motivated, and highly enthusiastic. They soak up learning opportunities as the earth soaks up rain following a lengthy dry spell. They deeply appreciate anything the leader does to support their learning.

Concepts of Learning

When the leader understands and applies the following concepts of learning, facilitation of learning increases significantly.

Learning is defined as a change in behavior. Many people falsely believe that if the teacher opens his or her mouth and articulately shares information, learning has occurred. Learning occurs only when a change in behavior takes place. Employees in an organization implementing teams can attend class after class of valuable information on how to make decisions and work as a team. But if their behavior does not change and they do not take the information back and apply it in the workplace, no learning has occurred.

Motivation of the learner is important. Adult learners are motivated by understanding and accepting the purposes of the learning situation. If a learner sees a direct need for the new knowledge or skill, the learner's readiness to learn greatly increases. When the learner perceives the new learning's usefulness and can readily identify the positive possible outcomes, learning is enhanced. In one organization an employee attending basic interpersonal skills development classes in preparation for the conversion to work teams was heard to say: "If I had known this ten years ago, my marriage wouldn't have ended in divorce." This participant was highly motivated to practice these skills in her current relationship.

Both learners and teachers are motivated by success. In planning early learning opportunities, there needs to be a fair certainty of success. For instance, if the leader is coaching a leader of a work team on conflict resolution skills, the teacher should start small. Perhaps the first situation should be a role play followed by facilitating the resolution of an intrateam conflict. If the first conflict that the team leader handles alone is a major conflict between teams in different departments, or between the team and a major customer (such as a physician), the stakes are too high.

Teacher acceptance is also reinforcing and motivational. Learners do better when they believe that the teacher accepts them unconditionally, in spite of the learner's need to gain competence in an area. The leader-teacher can demonstrate this through an objective and nonemotional acceptance of mistakes and by a sincere interest in helping the learner develop skills.

The learner's level of motivation almost completely determines the extent of learning. Adult learners make a choice about what they will learn. In many cases, the motivation is intrinsic and may be as simple as intellectual curiosity or the desire for increased personal competence.

Learning requires the learner's active participation. This increases the individual's commitment and level of ownership. When the learner participates, information becomes knowledge. Internalized by the learner, the knowledge begets new experiences and successes.

Learning is deepened when the learning situation provides the opportunity to apply learning in as realistic a situation as feasible. Using the skills and techniques in real-life situations greatly increases the learning, anchoring the learning in the individual's consciousness. The learner also modifies the skills and techniques based on their usefulness and gradually evolves beyond the original teaching.

Learning is enhanced when learners accept responsibility for their own learning. It is impossible to force someone to learn. The teacher's role is to make information and tools available, create the best learning situations possible, and provide the external motivation that encourages the learner during the process. Beyond this, the learner's responsibility is to take the ball and run.

Learning occurs on successively deeper levels. Sometimes highly expert teachers reduce their effectiveness because they try to give too much information at one time and move the learner too quickly. Of course, the higher the learner's development level, the faster he or she can go. In initial stages, the teacher delivers information in chunks, with the opportunity for the learner to practice and apply the new learning. A learner can be quite good at a skill yet not have the judgment and appropriate decision-making ability to support the skill.

Effective learning depends on repetition and feedback. Some adults are insulted when the teacher repeats a key piece of information, and they may feel impatient if they have heard it before. However, because every learner is an open system, the learner hearing the information a second time is a different person than when he or she first heard the information. The person has further experience and may actually be currently involved in a real-life situation that alters his or her perception of the information. Furthermore, conventional wisdom reports that we must hear something seven to eight times before it sinks in. The teacher's challenge is to find a multitude of ways to present the same information, changing and using new examples, and continually seeking ways to deliver the message through a variety of different channels.

Learners need the gift of feedback if they are to grow in their expertise. Feedback on performance gives the learner the opportunity to redirect and improve his or her dexterity with the knowledge. If the individual is not receiving clear, concise feedback on performance, he or she may think things are just fine when, in fact, there are problems.

Learning is stimulated by engaging a variety of senses. Drawing a picture, using colors, or listening to music all increase learning. Most teachers rely heavily on auditory stimulation and forget kinesthetic learning (having the person move) and the olfactory sense (smell).

An informal, friendly, and comfortable environment enhances learning. Atmosphere directly affects learning. If a room is too crowded, ventilation is poor, lights are low, or the air conditioning is too cold—any of these factors directly affects the learner's ability to listen and absorb information. Teachers who use embarrassment, humiliation, or shaming create a hostile environment in which learning revolves around how to avoid these adverse reactions rather than the positive development of beneficial skills.

For adults to learn new skills, the ideal is a risk-taking environment in which making a mistake is acceptable. In this environment mistakes are learning opportunities that increase the knowledge base and the wisdom of those involved. An optimal learning environment is one of mutual trust and high regard.

Teaching by Example

Another key principle of teaching is to teach by example. This is a way to demonstrate a skill and show how to do something. In addition, the leader's behavior demonstrates the leadership behaviors that the organization expects, desires, and rewards. Leaders are continually modeling behavior, which can create tremendous pressure for them. Nothing a leader does or says can escape the followers' notice. Every behavior and response, even a chance remark gives out a signal that a follower will pick up and pass on to others. Every action of the leader either validates or negates all the messages he or she has previously sent out. Followers can tell if a leader is sincere, honest, and congruent.

Some leaders are uncomfortable with this responsibility of influence and rail against the reality, claiming not to want to be a role model, not to want the pressure of followers watching their every move. The pressure to be a person of integrity, behaving consistently in accordance with stated beliefs, feels overwhelming at times. Some leaders complain: "I'm only human. . . . I can't be perfect." Or they think: *What I do in my private life is my own business; no one needs to know.* This is not to say that leaders do not need or have a right to privacy and time offstage. Leaders not only have this right but need to have private time to rejuvenate, relax, and not feel like someone is monitoring and evaluating their every move. However, the reality is that leadership increases the leader's visibility and vulnerability. When an individual moves out in front of the pack and picks up the reins of leadership, corresponding responsibilities appear. A primary responsibility is modeling expected behavior.

The reality of leading by example can be especially difficult if the leader is somewhat shy or reserved. Instead of focusing on the privacy that one has lost, perhaps the leader could consider this exposure as a gift. Most people perform better with a small amount of competition. When others are watching and expecting a high level of performance, we can feel the motivation to do better, to reach new heights of performance, and to excel at our task.

Conclusion

Exemplary leaders actively and intentionally participate in and contribute to their followers' growth and development. They coach for performance improvement by giving advice and instruction, encouraging discovery through guided discussions and actual experience, observing performance, and giving feedback. An involved leader positively influences followers by providing opportunities and engaging in teaching new skills. Followers grow and develop in and as a result of their relationship with an exemplary leader.

Conversation Points

1. How do you serve as a coach for others? Who have you coached in the past? What was your relationship like? What did you do successfully? What could you have done better?

2. Think about people who have been influential in your life, someone who has helped you develop new skills or served as your mentor. What were their coaching skills? What was most helpful to you?

3. Think about your personal and professional life. What motivates you? What internal motivators get you going in the morning? Are they present in all aspects of your life (personal, work, community)?

4. What examples of the self-fulfilling prophecy that you have seen have had positive effects? What are examples of those with negative or devastating effects?

5. What kind of behaviors are you emphasizing and rewarding in others around you? Is this the behavior you want to empha-

size? Are you inadvertently rewarding or recognizing any behaviors you don't want?

6. What elements of the coaching process do you use in your leadership practice? What are you very good at? Where do you need to improve?

7. What opportunities have you have been given in the past? How have they helped you grow? What are possibilities you have for sharing opportunities with others?

8. How do you incorporate the principles of adult learning in your interchanges when you teach others? How do you demonstrate respect for the people you are coaching? In what ways are the people you are coaching self-directed learners?

9. How do you feel about being a role model for others? Does this place pressure on you in any way? What examples of negative role modeling have you observed? What positive examples of role modeling have you seen?

8

Conclusion
Leading in the Future

Knowing is not enough, we must apply.
Willing is not enough, we must do.
                    Goethe *(from Brown,* On Success*)*

Health care has never been in greater need of exemplary leaders. It now finds itself at a major crossroads, with system integrations, mergers and acquisitions, hospital closures, reengineering and restructuring, downsizing and rightsizing, increased managed care penetration, new reimbursement models, increased regulatory constraints, accelerating consumer expectations, and intensified human relations issues all creating a tremendous demand for strong, skillful leaders. Even the leadership paradigm is shifting: the old command-and-control approach is simply no longer effective, and leaders at all levels need different skills for the future.

Some of these leadership skills or characteristics—integrity, a sense of mission, and a clear and inspiring vision—cannot be taught, except perhaps in life's classroom. The wisdom that comes from deep personal reflection and knowledge of what is most important brings a commitment to living by these values day to day, especially when we must make difficult choices that require courage and belief in ourselves. Most exemplary leaders have a desire to serve, to act in the interest of future generations. They function as true servant leaders, putting the needs of others first. And they believe they are in the right place at the right time. Fully engaged, with hearts committed, they clearly understand their purpose and envision a better future. A leader's vision creates the momentum that draws people to them and to their cause, to work together despite obstacles and challenges, to forge a new reality with hope and optimism for the future.

Although values, mission, and vision are not commonly taught through traditional methods, many leadership skills are—the numerous interpersonal skills that are this book's focus. Without excellent interpersonal skills and a high level of emotional intelligence, tomorrow's leaders cannot be successful. Paramount to this success are communication skills and the ability to form positive relationships with followers and gain their commitment to and engagement in a common purpose, as well as the ability to manage processes and develop others.

Relationships with followers greatly determine the degree of leaders' effectiveness. Trust, mutual respect, and open communication allow a leader's influence to flourish. Tomorrow's leaders collaborate and work with others in partnership. They thrive on interdependence and interconnections with other people.

Outstanding leaders recognize the distinction between compliance and commitment, and they want followers to fully engage with their hearts. These leaders are people who are not afraid to express their deeply held values and cherished beliefs, creating a collective sense of mission and a shared vision—a powerful force for transformation.

Exceptional leaders are master communicators. They constantly reflect on and evaluate their effectiveness, seeking to expand their verbal and nonverbal skills. They use anecdotes, analogies, and metaphors and evoke powerful symbols to communicate the organization's most important and deeply held values. They work diligently to overcome barriers to effective communication, becoming versatile in interpreting differences in tribal language, gender, and style.

Exceptional leaders also understand and effectively facilitate process so that the processes they and their followers engage in are meaningful. They recognize and knowledgeably apply the sequential steps of a process, allowing it to unfold within its natural time frame; and they develop sound judgment that alerts them to the need to nudge a process along. As process facilitators, these leaders demonstrate by example how to empower others, resolve conflict, lead a problem-solving process, reach decisions, create teams, and manage change. They use their judgment to determine when to use appreciative inquiry or a traditional problem-solving process. They recognize when the issue before them is a polarity to manage rather than a problem to solve.

And finally, extraordinary leaders constantly seek opportunities to develop others. They do this by intentional and proactive coaching, facilitating the development of followers' skills by giving instruction and advice, and by encouraging discovery through guided discussions and hands-on experiences. They observe performance and provide honest, direct, and timely feedback. These leaders diligently seek to provide opportunities for followers and constantly teach and share their knowledge with them. Leaders themselves are continual learners, thriving among colleagues who are also continual learners.

Each of these competencies is essential, and without the complete package, influence is difficult to attain. No competency is easy to develop, however, often requiring years of experience taking risks and making mistakes, trying again and yet again. It is helpful to remember Brown's (1994, p. 78) sage advice: "Remember that overnight success usually takes about fifteen years."

Society cannot afford the cost and consequence of weak leadership in health care. Health care leaders today are stewards for the future, and we will build healthier communities only through full collaboration of the health care system, local government, civic leaders, and federal legislators.

Leadership development is an intensely personal, lifelong journey. Warren Bennis (1989, p. 112) puts it particularly well: "No leader sets out to be a leader. People set out to live their lives, expressing themselves fully. When that expression is of value, they become leaders. So the point is not to become a leader. The point is to become yourself, to use yourself completely—all your skills, gifts, and energies—in order to make your vision manifest. You must withhold nothing. You must, in sum, become the person you started out to be, and to enjoy the process of becoming."

This journey is not an easy one, and it may help to reflect on the following story of a bedridden gentleman. One day this man noticed a caterpillar crawling along the windowsill next to his bed. To his delight, it stopped in the corner and began spinning a cocoon. The man was excited because he knew eventually he would watch a beautiful butterfly emerge. Weeks later he noticed movement in the cocoon. Eager to behold the transformation to a new butterfly, he watched and waited. But the struggle continued. Growing impatient, the man decided to help speed the labor along. He opened the window, and then he gently picked up the cocoon. Carefully opening it, he was enchanted to see the new butterfly emerge. It staggered a few steps and, to the man's dismay, fell over and died. What the man failed to realize is that it is in the efforts to emerge from the cocoon that a butterfly gains enough strength to fly away.

Like the difficulties for a butterfly emerging from a cocoon, the inherent struggles of leading build the strength to lead and meet the challenges of today's health care organizations. Leadership is not glamorous; it is hard work. Doing the right thing even at high personal cost takes courage, and it takes a belief in something bigger than oneself. It takes the optimism and hope to dream about the wonderful possibilities, although dreaming is not enough. Perseverance and dedication are needed to implement the strategies that will transform present reality into that desired future. Leadership is an opportunity and a gift to those privileged to accept its challenges.

References

AbuAlRub, R. F. "Job Stress, Job Performance, and Social Support Among Hospital Nurses." *Journal of Nursing Scholarship*, 2004, 36(1), 73–78.

Ackoff, R., Finnel, E., and Gharajedaghi, J. *A Guide to Controlling Your Corporation's Future.* New York: Wiley, 1984.

Adams, D. C. "False Metaphors." *Hospitals & Health Networks*, Nov. 5, 1995, pp. 42–44.

Adams, J. L. *The Care and Feeding of Ideas: A Guide to Encouraging Creativity.* Reading, Mass.: Addison-Wesley, 1986.

Aiken, L. H., Clarke, S. P., and Stone, D. M. "Hospital Staffing, Organization, and Quality of Care: Cross-National Findings." *Nursing Outlook*, 2002, 50(5), 187–194.

American Hospital Association. "Staffing Watch." *Hospitals & Health Networks*, Sept. 2001, p. 22.

American Nurses Association (ANA). *Nursing World Health and Safety Survey.* Washington, D.C.: Nursing World, 2001.

Anderson, P. *Great Quotes from Great Leaders.* Lombard, Ill.: Celebrating Excellence, 1990.

Ankario, L. Quoted in "Know How to Lead." *Tampa Tribune*, March 3, 1993.

Annas, G. J. "Beyond the Military and Market Metaphors." *Healthcare Forum Journal*, 1996 (May/June), 30–34.

Annison, M. "Leadership." *Westrend Letter*, 1994 (June), 1–4.

Annison, M. Keynote address at the Florida Hospital Association annual meeting, Orlando, Fla., Nov. 13, 1997.

Aronson, E. *The Social Animal.* 7th ed. New York: Freeman, 1995.

Baggs, J. G., and Schmitt, M. H. "Collaboration Between Nurses and Physicians." *Image: Journal of Nursing Scholarship*, 1988, 20(3), 145–149.

Bandler, R., and Grinder, J. *From Frogs into Princes: Neuro-Linguistic Programming*. Moab, Utah: Real People Press, 1979.

Bardwick, J. M. "Emotional Leaders." *Executive Excellence*, 1996 (Apr.), 13–14.

Barker, J. A. *The Power of Vision*. Burnsville, Minn.: Charthouse Learning Corporation, 1990. Videotape.

Barker, J. A. *Paradigms: The Business of Discovering the Future*. New York: HarperCollins, 1992.

Barney, S. M. "Radical Change: One Solution to the Nursing Shortage." *Journal of Healthcare Management*, 2002, 47(4), 220–223.

Barrett, F. J. "Creating Appreciative Learning Cultures." *Organization Dynamics*, 1995, 24, 36–49.

Batcheller, J., and others. "A Practice Model for Patient Safety: The Value of the Experienced Registered Nurse." *Journal of Nursing Administration*, 2004, 34(4), 200–205.

Becker, H. S. "Notes on the Concept of Commitment." *American Journal of Sociology*, 1960, 66, 32–40.

Beckhard, R., and Pritchard, W. *Changing the Essence: The Art of Creating and Leading Fundamental Change in Organizations*. San Francisco: Jossey-Bass, 1992.

Benner, P. *From Novice to Expert*. Menlo Park, Calif.: Addison-Wesley, 1984.

Bennis, W. *On Becoming a Leader*. Reading, Mass.: Addison-Wesley, 1989.

Bennis, W., and Nanus, B. *Leaders: The Strategies for Taking Charge*. New York: HarperCollins, 1985.

Berry, L. L. "Qualities of Leadership." *Retailing Issues Letter*, 1992, 4(1), 1–4.

Blanchard, K. H., and Johnson, S. *The One-Minute Manager*. New York: Berkley, 1981.

Block, P. *The Empowered Manager: Positive Political Skills at Work*. San Francisco: Jossey-Bass, 1987.

Blouin, A., and Brent, N. "Strategic Partnering: Clinical and Risk Management Concerns." *Journal of Nursing Administration*, 1997, 27(6), 10–13.

Bossidy, L., and Charan, R. *Execution: The Discipline of Getting Things Done*. New York: Crown Business, 2002.

Bowcutt, M. "Maintaining a Balance." *Nurse Leader*, 2004 (Apr.), 25–27.

Brickman, P., Wortman, C. B., and Sorrentino, R. (eds.). *Commitment, Conflict, and Caring*. Englewood Cliffs, N.J.: Prentice Hall, 1987.

Bridges, W. *Transitions: Making Sense of Life's Changes*. Reading, Mass.: Addison-Wesley, 1980.

Bridges, W. *Surviving Corporate Transition*. Mill Valley, Calif.: William Bridges & Associates, 1988.

Bridges, W. *Managing Transitions: Making the Most of Change*. Mill Valley, Calif.: William Bridges & Associates, 1991.

Bridges, W. *Participant's Guide: Managing Organizational Transitions*. Mill Valley, Calif.: William Bridges & Associates, 1992.

Bridges, W. *JobShift*. Mill Valley, Calif.: William Bridges & Associates, 1994a.

Bridges, W. "The End of the Job." *Fortune*, Sept. 19, 1994b, pp. 62–74.

Bridges, W. "Leadership and the De-Jobbed Organization." *Organizations in Transition*, 1995, 8(2), 5.

Brown, H. J., Jr. *Life's Little Treasure Book on Success*. Nashville, Tenn.: Rutledge Hill Press, 1994.

Buckingham, M., and Coffman, C. *First, Break All the Rules: What the World's Greatest Managers Do Differently*. New York: Simon & Schuster, 1999.

Burns, B. M. *Leadership*. New York: HarperCollins, 1978.

Byers, J. F., and White, S. V. (eds.). *Patient Safety: Principles and Practice*. New York: Springer, 2004.

Byrne, J. A. "How to Lead Now: Getting Extraordinary Performance When You Can't Pay for It." *Fast Company*, 2003 (Aug.), 62–70.

Campbell, R., and Inguagiato, R. "The Power of Listening." *Physician Executive*, 1994, 20(9), 35–37.

Chaleff, I. "Effective Leadership." *Executive Excellence*, 1996 (Apr.), 16–17.

Chaleff, I. "The Groupthink Challenge." *Team Management Briefings*, 1997 (June), 4.

Champy, J. "The Hidden Qualities of Great Leaders." *Fast Company*, 2003 (Nov.), 135.

Chawla, S., and Renesch, J. (eds.). *Learning Organizations: Developing Cultures for Tomorrow's Workplace*. Portland, Oreg.: Productivity Press, 1995.

Cherniss, C., and Goleman, D. (eds.). *The Emotionally Intelligent Workplace: How to Select for, Measure, and Improve Emotional Intelligence in Individuals, Groups, and Organizations*. San Francisco: Jossey-Bass, 2001.

Ciancutti, A., and Steding, T. L. *Built on Trust: Gaining Competitive Advantage in Any Organization*. Chicago: Contemporary Books, 2001.

Clancy, T. "The Art of Decision-Making." *Journal of Nursing Administration*, 2003, 33(6), 343–349.

Clark, M. "Metaphorically Speaking." *Healthcare Forum Journal*, 1996 (May/June), 20–27.

Clarke-Epstein, C. "Truth in Feedback." *Training and Development*, 2002 (Nov.), 78–80.

Coens, T., and Jenkins, M. *Abolishing Performance Appraisals: Why They Backfire and What to Do Instead*. San Francisco: Berrett-Koehler, 2000.

Collins, J. *Good to Great: Why Some Companies Make the Leap . . . and Others Don't*. New York: HarperCollins, 2001.

Collins, S. *Stillpoint: The Dance of Selfcaring, Selfhealing*. Fort Worth, Tex.: TLC Productions, 1992.

Connor, D. *Managing at the Speed of Change: How Resilient Managers Succeed and Prosper Where Others Fail*. New York: Villard Books, 1993.

Cooper, R. K. "21st Leadership: Excelling Under Pressure." Paper presented at a meeting of the American Organization of Nurse Executives, Charlotte, N.C., March 1999.

Covey, S. *The Seven Habits of Highly Effective People: Restoring the Character Ethic*. New York: Simon & Schuster, 1989.

Covey, S. *Principle-Centered Leadership*. New York: Simon & Schuster, 1990.

Covey, S., Merrill, A. R., and Merrill, R. R. *First Things First*. New York: Simon & Schuster, 1994.

Cox, S., Manion, J., and Miller, D. *Nature's Wisdom in the Workplace: Managing Energy in Today's Health Care Organization*. Bloomington, Minn.: Synergy Press, 2005.

Creative Healthcare Management. *Leaders Empower Staff Participant Manual*. Minneapolis: Creative Healthcare Management, 1994.

Csikszentmihalyi, M. *Flow: The Psychology of Optimal Experience*. New York: HarperCollins, 1990.

Csikszentmihalyi, M. *Finding Flow: The Psychology of Engagement with Everyday Life*. New York: Basic Books, 1997.

Csikszentmihalyi, M. *Good Business: Leadership, Flow, and the Making of Meaning*. New York: Penguin Putnam Books, 2003.

Curtin, L. "Blessed Are the Flexible." *Nursing Management*, 1995, 26(3), 7–8.

Delbecq, A. L., and VandeVen, A. H. "A Group Process Model for Problem Identification and Program Planning." *Journal of Applied Behavioral Science*, 1971, 7, 466–494.

de Man, H. *Joy in Work*. London: George Allen & Unwin, 1929.

DePree, M. *Leadership Is an Art*. New York: Bantam, Doubleday, 1989.

Drucker, P. *Managing for the Future: The 1990s and Beyond*. New York: Penguin Books, 1992.

Eisler, R. *The Chalice and the Blade: Our History, Our Future*. New York: Harper-Collins, 1987.

Eisler, R., and Loye, D. *The Partnership Way: New Tools for Living and Learning*. 2nd ed. Brandon, Vt.: Holistic Education Press, 1998.

Fagiano, D. "Designating a Leader." *Management Review*, 1994 (Mar.), 4.

Fielden, J. "What Do You Mean I Can't Write?" *Journal of Nursing Administration*, 1981, *11*(3), 42–47.

Fields, M., and Zwisler, S. "Walk in Balance: Returning to the Self." *Nurse Leader*, 2004 (Apr.), 44–45.

Flower, J. "The Chasm Between Management and Leadership." *Healthcare Forum Journal*, 1990, *33*(4), 59–62.

Flower, J. "Being Effective." *Healthcare Forum Journal*, 1991, *34*(3), 52–57.

Flower, J. "Job Shift." *Healthcare Forum Journal*, 1997, *40*(1), 14–21.

Frederickson, B. "What Good are Positive Emotions?" Authentic Happiness Coaching seminar, June 10, 2004.

Freshwater, D. "Reflective Practice: A Tool for Developing Clinical Leadership." *Reflections on Nursing Leadership*, 2004 (2nd qtr.), 20–26.

Frick, D., and Spears, L. (eds.). *On Becoming a Servant-Leader: The Private Writings of Robert K. Greenleaf*. San Francisco: Jossey-Bass, 1996.

Gelinas, L., and Bohlen, C. *Tomorrow's Work Force: A Strategic Approach*. Irving, Tex.: Voluntary Hospitals of America, 2002.

Gibson, C. "A Concept Analysis of Empowerment." *Journal of Advanced Nursing*, 1991, *16*, 354–361.

Gilligan, C. *In a Different Voice: Psychological Theory of Woman's Development*. Cambridge, Mass.: Harvard University Press, 1982.

Goleman, D. *Emotional Intelligence: Why It Can Matter More Than IQ*. New York: Bantam Books, 1994.

Goleman, D., Boyatzis, R., and McKee, A. *Primal Leadership: Realizing the Power of Emotional Intelligence*. Boston: Harvard Business School Press, 2002.

Gray, J. *Men Are from Mars, Women Are from Venus*. New York: HarperCollins, 1992.

Grossman, R. J. "The Looming Crisis: Health Care Organizations Are Behind Other Industries in Cultivating Tomorrow's Leaders." *Health Forum Journal*, 1999 (Nov./Dec.), 18–25.

Heenan, D. A., and Bennis, W. *Co-Leaders: The Power of Great Partnerships*. New York: Wiley, 1999.

Heifetz, R. A., and Laurie, D. L. "The Work of Leadership." *Harvard Business Review*, 1997 (Jan./Feb.), 124–134.

Henry, B., and LeClair, H. "Language, Leadership, and Power." *Journal of Nursing Administration*, 1987, *17*(1), 19–24.

Hersey, P., and Blanchard, K. H. *Management of Organizational Behavior: Utilizing Human Resources*. 6th ed. Englewood, N.J.: Prentice Hall, 1993.

Hesselbein, F., Goldsmith, M., and Beckhard, R. (eds.). *The Leader of the Future*. San Francisco: Jossey-Bass, 1996.

Huey, J. "The New Post-Heroic Leadership." *Fortune*, Feb. 21, 1994, pp. 45–50.

Iverson, R., and Buttigieg, D. "Affective, Normative and Continuance Commitment: Can the 'Right Kind' of Commitment Be Managed?" *Journal of Management Studies*, 1999, 36(3), 307–333.

Iyengar, S. S., and Lepper, M. R. "Rethinking the Value of Choice: A Cultural Perspective on Intrinsic Motivation." *Journal of Personality and Social Psychology*, 1999, 76(3), 349–366.

Johns, C. "Becoming a Transformational Leader Through Reflection." *Reflections on Nursing Leadership*, 2004 (2nd qtr.), 24–26.

Johnson, B. *Polarity Management: Identifying and Managing Unsolvable Problems*. Amherst, Mass.: HRD Press, 1996.

Johnson, J. A. "Warren Bennis, Chairman, The Leadership Institute" *Journal of Healthcare Management*, 1998, 43(4), 293–296.

Kanter, R. M. *Commitment and Community: Communes and Utopias in Sociological Perspective*. Cambridge, Mass.: Harvard University Press, 1972.

Kanter, R. M. *On the Frontiers of Management*. Middlebury, Vt.: Soundview Executive Book Summaries, 1997.

Katzenbach, J. R., and Smith, D. K. *The Wisdom of Teams: Creating the High-Performance Organization*. Boston: Harvard Business School Press, 1993.

Kaye, B., and Jordan-Evans, S. "Retention in Tough Times." *Training & Development*, 2002 (Jan.), 32–37.

Knowles, M. *The Modern Practice of Adult Education: Andragogy Versus Pedagogy*. Chicago: Association Press, 1970.

Kostner, J. *Knights of the TeleRound Table*. New York: Warner Books, 1994.

Kouzes, J. W., and Posner, B. Z. *The Leadership Challenge*. 2nd ed. San Francisco: Jossey-Bass, 1987.

Kouzes, J. W., and Posner, B. Z. "The Credibility Factor." *Healthcare Forum Journal*, 1993a (July/Aug.), 16–24.

Kouzes, J. W., and Posner, B. Z. *The Credibility Factor*. San Francisco: Jossey-Bass, 1993b.

Kouzes, J. W., and Posner, B. Z. *The Leadership Challenge*. 3rd ed. San Francisco: Jossey-Bass, 2002.

Kouzes, J. W., and Posner, B. Z. *Encouraging the Heart: A Leader's Guide to Rewarding and Recognizing Others*. San Francisco: Jossey-Bass, 2003.

Kowalski, K., and Yoder-Wise, P. "Five Cs of Leadership." *Nurse Leader*, 2003 (Sept./Oct.), 26–31.

Kraemer, H. "Keeping It Simple." *Health Forum Journal*, 2003 (summer), 16–20.

Larson, C. E., and LaFasto, F. *TeamWork: What Must Go Right/What Can Go Wrong*. Newbury Park, Calif.: Sage, 1989.

Larson, P., and William, L. "Striving for Balance: A Thing of the Past?" *Nurse Leader*, 2004 (Apr.), 37–39.

Leander, W., Shortridge, D., and Watson, P. *Patients First*. Chicago: Health Care Administration Press, 1996.

Lencioni, P. *The Five Dysfunctions of a Team: A Leadership Fable*. San Francisco: Jossey-Bass, 2002.

Loehr, J., and Schwartz, T. *The Power of Full Engagement: Managing Energy, Not Time, Is the Key to High Performance and Personal Renewal*. New York: Free Press, 2003.

Lorimer, W., and Manion, J. "Team-Based Organizations: Leading the Essential Transformation." *Patient Focused Care Association Review*, 1996 (summer), 15–19.

Ludema, J. D., Cooperrider, D. L., and Barrett, F. J. "Appreciative Inquiry: The Power of the Unconditional Positive Question." In P. Reason and H. Bradbury (eds.), *Handbook of Action Research*. London: Sage, 2000.

Lydon, J. E., and Zanna, M. P. "Commitment in the Face of Adversity: A Value-Affirmation Approach." *Journal of Personality and Social Psychology*, 1990, 58(6), 1040–1047.

Makin, P. J., Cooper, C. L., and Cox, C. J. *Organizations and the Psychological Contract: Managing People at Work*. Westport, Conn.: Quorum Books, 1996.

Manion, J. "Professional Collaboration: More Than a Committee Structure." *Nursing Options*, 1989, 1(4), 9–12.

Manion, J. *Change from Within: Nurse Intrapreneurs as Health Care Innovators*. Kansas City, Mo.: American Nurses Association, 1990.

Manion, J. "Chaos or Transformation? Managing Innovation." *Journal of Nursing Administration*, 1993, 23(5), 41–48.

Manion, J. "Managing Change: The Leadership Challenge of the 1990s." *Seminars for Nurse Managers*, 1994, 2(4), 203–208.

Manion, J. "Understanding the Seven Stages of Change." *American Journal of Nursing*, 1995, 95(4), 41–43.

Manion, J. "Teams 101: The Manager's Role." *Seminars for Nurse Managers*, 1997, 5(1), 31–38.

Manion, J. "Building Commitment in Today's Workforce." *Home Care Provider*, 2000a (Aug.), 130–131.

Manion, J. "Retaining Current Leaders: A Gold Mine in Your Back Yard." *Health Forum Journal*, 2000b, *43*(5), 24–27.

Manion, J. "Joy at Work: As Experience, As Expressed" Unpublished doctoral dissertation, Fielding Graduate Institute, 2002a.

Manion, J. "Emergence of the Free Agent Workforce." *Nursing Administration Quarterly*, 2002b, *26*(5), 68–78.

Manion, J. "Joy at Work: Creating a Positive Workplace." *Journal of Nursing Administration*, 2003, *33*(12), 652–659.

Manion, J. "Strengthening Organizational Commitment: Understanding the Concept as a Basis for Creating Effective Workforce Retention Strategies." *Health Care Manager*, 2004a, *23*(2), 167–176.

Manion, J. "Nurture a Culture of Retention: Front-line Nurse Leaders Share Perceptions Regarding What Makes—or Breaks—a Flourishing Nursing Environment." *Nursing Management*, 2004b, *35*(4), 28–39.

Manion, J., and Bartholomew, K. "Community in the Workplace: A Proven Retention Strategy." *Journal of Nursing Administration*, 2004, *34*(1), 46–53.

Manion, J., Lorimer, W., and Leander, W. *Team-Based Health Care Organizations: Blueprint for Success*. Gaithersburg, Md.: Aspen, 1996.

Manion, J., Sieg, M. J., and Watson, P. "Managerial Partnerships: The Wave of the Future?" *Journal of Nursing Administration*, 1998, *28*(4), 47–55.

Manion, J., and Watson, P. "Developing Team-Based Patient Care Through Reengineering." In S. S. Blanchett and D. L. Flarey (eds.), *Reengineering Nursing and Health Care*. Gaithersburg, Md.: Aspen, 1995.

Markels, A. "Memo 4/8/97, FYI: Messages Inundate Offices." *Wall Street Journal*, Apr. 8, 1997, p. B1.

Maun, C. Speech for the Maryland Healthcare Institute, Baltimore, June 1, 2004.

Maxwell, J. "Inspiration Point." *Nurse Leader*, 2003, *1*(5), 8.

Mayer, J. D., Salovey, P., and Caruso, D. R. "Models of Human Intelligence." In R. J. Sternberg (ed.), *Handbook of Human Intelligence*. 2nd ed. New York: Cambridge University Press, 2000.

Mayer, R., and Schoorman, D. "Differentiating Antecedents of Organizational Commitment." *Journal of Organizational Behavior*, 1998, *19*(1), 15–28.

McCarthy, D. *The Loyalty Link*. New York: Wiley, 1997.

McConnell, C. R. "Interpersonal Skills: What They Are, How to Improve

Them, and How to Apply Them." *Health Care Manager*, 2004, *23*(2), 177–187.

McDonald, T. "Send Clear Messages." *Team Management Briefings*, 1997, 4.

McGinnis, A. L. *Bringing Out the Best in People*. Minneapolis: Augsburg Fortress, 1985.

McNeese-Smith, D., and Crook, M. "Nursing Values and a Changing Nursing Workforce." *Journal of Nursing Administration*, 2003, *33*(5), 260–270.

Melrose, K. "Leader as Servant." *Executive Excellence*, 1996, *13*(4), 20.

Meyer, J., and others. "Organizational Commitment and Job Performance: It's the Nature of the Commitment That Counts." *Journal of Applied Psychology*, 1989, *74*(1), 152–156.

Meyer, J. P., and Allen, N. J. "Testing the 'Side-Bet Theory' of Organizational Commitment: Some Methodological Considerations." *Journal of Applied Psychology*, 1984, *69*(3), 372–378.

Miller, D., and Manthey, M. "Empowerment Through Levels of Authority." *Journal of Nursing Administration*, 1994, *24*(7), 23.

Minor, M. *Coaching and Counseling: A Practical Guide for Managers*. Menlo Park, Calif.: Crisp, 1989.

Mintzberg, H. *The Nature of Managerial Work*. Englewood Cliffs, N.J.: Prentice Hall, 1980.

Morris, D. *Manwatching: A Field Guide to Human Behavior*. New York: Abrams, 1979.

Mycek, S. "Leadership for a Healthy Twenty-First Century." *Healthcare Forum Journal*, 1998, *41*(4), 26–30.

Neuhauser, P. C. *Tribal Warfare in Organizations*. Cambridge, Mass.: Ballinger, 1988.

Nierenberg, J., and Ross, I. *Women and the Art of Negotiating*. New York: Simon & Schuster, 1985.

Noer, D. M. *Healing the Wounds: Overcoming the Trauma of Layoffs and Revitalizing Downsized Organizations*. San Francisco: Jossey-Bass, 1993.

Oakley, E., and Krug, D. *Enlightened Leadership*. New York: Simon & Schuster, 1993.

O'Dooley, P. *Flight Plan for Living: The Art of Self Encouragement*. New York: Master Media, 1992.

Parker, G. "Teamwork and Team Players." *Team Management Briefings*, 1997, *5*(5), 8.

Peck, M. S. *The Road Less Traveled*. New York: Simon & Schuster, 1978.

Perot, R. "Caring Leaders." *Executive Excellence*, 1996 (Apr.), 6–7.

Pesmen, S. *Orlando Sentinel*, May 27, 1990, p. E21.

Peters, T. *Thriving on Chaos*. New York: HarperCollins, 1987.

Peters, T., and Austin, N. *A Passion for Excellence*. New York: Random House, 1985.

Phillips, D. *Lincoln on Leadership: Executive Strategies for Tough Times*. New York: Warner Books, 1992.

Pinchot, G., and Pinchot, E. "Creating Space for Many Leaders." *Executive Excellence*, 1996a, *13*(4), 17–18.

Pinchot, G., and Pinchot, E. *The Intelligent Organization: Engaging the Talent and Initiative of Everyone in the Workplace*. San Francisco: Berrett-Koehler, 1996b.

Porter-O'Grady, T., and Malloch, K. *Quantum Leadership: A Textbook of New Leadership*. Boston: Jones and Bartlett, 2003.

Post, N. *Working Balance: Energy Management for Personal and Professional Well-Being*. Philadelphia: Post Enterprises, 1989.

Productivity and the Self-Fulfilling Prophecy: The Pygmalion Effect. (2nd ed.) Carlsbad, Calif.: CRM Films, 1997.

Quotable Women: A Collection of Shared Thoughts. Philadelphia: Running Press, 1989.

Reina, D. S., and Reina, M. L. *Trust and Betrayal in the Workplace: Building Effective Relationships in Your Organization*. San Francisco: Berrett-Koehler, 1999.

Rogers, R. "The Psychological Contract of Trust." *Executive Excellence*, 1994 (July), 6.

Seashore, C., Seashore, E., and Weinberg, G. *What Did You Say? The Art of Giving and Receiving Feedback*. Columbia, Md.: Bingham House Books, 1999.

Seligman, M. E. *Authentic Happiness: Using the New Positive Psychology to Realize Your Potential for Lasting Fulfillment*. New York: Simon & Schuster, 2002.

Senge, P. M. *The Fifth Discipline: The Art and Practice of the Learning Organization*. New York: Doubleday, 1990.

Senge, P. M. "Leading Learning Organizations." *Executive Excellence*, 1996 (Apr.), 10–11.

Shula, D., and Blanchard, K. H. *Everyone's a Coach*. Grand Rapids, Mich.: Zondervan, 1995.

Smith, S. S. "The Power of Praise." *The Costco Connection*, 2003 (Mar.), 16–18.

Stacey, R. *Managing the Unknowable: Strategic Boundaries Between Order and Chaos in Organizations*. San Francisco: Jossey-Bass, 1992.

Tannen, D. *Talking from 9 to 5*. New York: Avon, 1994.

Tarkenton, F., with Tuleja, T. *How to Motivate People*. New York: HarperCollins, 1986.

Taylor, B. J. "Improving Communication Through Practical Reflection." *Reflections on Nursing Leadership*, 2004 (2nd qtr.), 28–38.

Thomas, K. W. *Intrinsic Motivation at Work: Building Energy and Commitment*. San Francisco: Berrett-Koehler, 2000.

Tichy, N., with Cardwell, N. *The Cycle of Leadership: How Great Leaders Teach Their Companies to Win*. New York: HarperCollins, 2002.

Trigg, R. *Reason and Commitment*. Cambridge: University Press, 1973.

Ulreich, S. "Balancing Life—In Heels and a Suit." *Nurse Leader*, 2004 (Apr.), 32–35.

Unruh, L. "Impact of Nurse Staffing on Patient Safety." In J. F. Byers and S. White (eds.), *Patient Safety: Principles and Practice*. New York: Springer, 2004.

Van Allen, L. "Permission to Balance Work and Life." *Nurse Leader*, 2004 (Apr.), 40–43.

Vance, M. *Creative Thinking*. Chicago: Nightingale-Conant Corporation, 1982. Audiotape series.

Von Oech, R. *A Whack on the Side of the Head: How to Unlock Your Mind for Innovation*. New York: Warner Books, 1983.

Von Oech, R. *A Kick in the Seat of the Pants: Using Your Explorer, Artist, Judge, and Warrior to Be More Creative*. New York: Harper & Row, 1986.

Waterman, R. H. *The Renewal Factor: How the Best Get and Keep the Competitive Edge*. New York: Bantam Books, 1987.

Waterman, R. H. *Adhocracy: The Power to Change*. New York: Norton, 1992.

Wesorick, B. "Twenty-First Century Leadership Challenge: Creating and Sustaining Healthy Healing Work Cultures and Integrated Service at the Point of Care." *Nursing Administration Quarterly*, 2002, 26(5), 18–32.

Wheatley, M. J. *Leadership and the New Science*. San Francisco: Berrett-Koehler, 1992.

Wiener, Y. "Commitment in Organizations." *Academy of Management Review*, 1982, 7(3), 418–428.

Wilson, J., George, J., and Wellins, R. *Leadership Trapeze: Strategies for Leadership in Team-Based Organizations*. San Francisco: Jossey-Bass, 1994.

Wycoff, J. *Mindmapping: Your Personal Guide to Exploring Creativity and Problem-Solving*. New York: Berkley, 1991.

Zemke, R. "The Corporate Coach." *Training*, 1996, 33(12), 24–33.

Zemke, R. "Problem-Solving Is the Problem: Don't Fix That Company." *Training*, 1999, 36(6), 26–33.

Additional Reading

Abbasi, S., and Hollman, K. "Self-Managed Teams: The Productivity Break-through of the 1990s." *Journal of Managerial Psychology,* 1994, 9(7), 25–30.

American Hospital Association. *In Our Hands: How Hospital Leaders Can Build a Thriving Workforce.* Chicago: American Hospital Association, 2002.

Argyris, C. "Good Communication That Blocks Learning." *Harvard Business Review,* 1994 (July/Aug.), 77–85.

Bardwick, J. M. *Danger in the Comfort Zone.* New York: American Management Association, 1991.

Becker-Reems, E. D. *Self-Managed Work Teams in Health Care Organizations.* Chicago: American Hospital Association, 1994.

Belasco, J. A. *Teaching the Elephant to Dance: Empowering Change in Your Organization.* New York: Crown, 1990.

Belasco, J. A., and Stayer, R. C. *Flight of the Buffalo: Soaring to Excellence, Learning to Let Employees Lead.* New York: Warner Books, 1993.

Blancett, S. S., and Flarey, D. L. *Reengineering Nursing and Health Care: The Handbook for Organizational Transformation.* Gaithersburg, Md.: Aspen, 1995.

Blanchard, K., and Bowles, S. *Raving Fans: A Revolutionary Approach to Customer Service.* New York: Morrow, 1993.

Blanchard, K., Oncken, W., and Burrows, H. *The One-Minute Manager Meets the Monkey.* New York: Morrow, 1989.

Bohan, G. P. "Building a High-Performance Team." *Health Care Supervisor,* 1990, 8(4), 15–21.

Bolman, L. G., and Deal, T. E. *Leading with Soul: An Uncommon Journey of Spirit.* San Francisco: Jossey-Bass, 1995.

351

Buggie, F. "Expert Innovation Teams: A New Way to Increase Productivity Dramatically." *Planning Review*, 1995, *23*(4), 26–31.

Byham, W. C., with Cox, J. *Zapp! The Lightning of Empowerment: How to Improve Productivity, Quality, and Employee Satisfaction*. New York: Harmony Books, 1988.

Carr, C. "Planning Priorities for Empowered Teams." *Journal of Business Strategy*, 1992, *13*(5), 43–47.

Cooperrider, D., and Srivastva, S. (eds.). *Appreciative Management and Leadership: The Power of Positive Thought and Action in Organizations*. San Francisco: Jossey-Bass, 1990.

Curtin, L. "The Gold Collar Leader . . . ?" *Nursing Management*, 1995, *26*(10), 7–8.

Dailey, R., Young, F., and Barr, C. "Empowering Middle Managers in Hospitals with Team-Based Problem-Solving." *Health Care Management Review*, 1991, *16*(2), 55–63.

DePree, M. *Leadership Jazz*. New York: Doubleday, 1992.

Distefano, S. M., and Bledsoe, D. N. "A Balanced Approach to Leadership." *Nurse Leader*, 2003 (Sept./Oct.), 32–35.

Drucker, P. *The New Realities*. New York: HarperCollins, 1989.

Dubnicki, C. "Building High-Performance Management Teams: The Shape of Things to Come." *Healthcare Forum Journal*, 1991, *34*(5), 10–11.

Dubnicki, C., and Limburg, W. "How Do Healthcare Teams Measure Up?" *Healthcare Forum Journal*, 1991, *34*(5), 10–11.

Dumaine, B. "The Trouble with Teams." *Fortune*, Sept. 5, 1994, pp. 86–92.

Duncan, E. A., and Warden, G. L. "Influential Leadership and Change Environment: The Role Leaders Play in the Growth and Development of the People They Lead." *Journal of Healthcare Management*, 1999, *44*(4), 225–226.

Dychtwald, K., with Flower, J. *Age Wave: How the Most Important Trend of Our Time Will Change Your Future*. New York: Bantam Books, 1990.

Filson, B. "The New Leadership." *Hospitals & Health Networks*, Sept. 5, 1994, p. 76.

Fisher, K. *Leading Self-Directed Work Teams: A Guide to Developing New Team Leadership Skills*. New York: McGraw-Hill, 1993.

Garber, P. R. *Coaching Self-Directed Work Teams: Building Winning Teams in Today's Changing Workplace*. King of Prussia, Pa.: Organization Design and Development, 1993.

Geber, B. "From Manager into Coach." *Training*, 1992, *29*(2), 25–31.

Glaser, R. *Moving Your Team Toward Self-Management.* King of Prussia, Pa.: Organization Design and Development, 1990.

Glaser, R. *Facilitating Self-Managing Teams.* King of Prussia, Pa.: Organization Design and Development, 1991a.

Glaser, R. *Learning to Be a Self-Managing Team.* King of Prussia, Pa.: Organization Design and Development, 1991b.

Glaser, R. *Classic Readings in Self-Managing Teamwork.* King of Prussia, Pa.: Organization Design and Development, 1992.

Glines, D. "Do You Work in a Zoo?" *Executive Excellence,* 1994 (Oct.), 12–13.

Goldberg, B. "Team Rewards and Team Benefits." *Executive Excellence,* 1995 (June), 14–15.

Goman, C. K. *Adapting to Change: Making It Work for You.* Menlo Park, Calif.: Crisp, 1992.

Goodemote, E. "Managing in the Next Decade: A New Set of Skills for Nurse Managers." *Seminars for Nurse Managers,* 1995, *3*(2), 84–88.

Gummer, B. "Post-Industrial Management: Teams, Self-Management, and the New Interdependence." *Administration in Social Work,* 1988, *12*(3), 117–132.

Hamilton, J. "Toppling the Power of the Pyramid." *Hospitals,* Jan. 5, 1993, p. 33.

Hammond, S. A. *The Thin Book of Appreciative Inquiry.* 2nd ed. Plano, Tex.: Thin Book, 1998.

Hammond, S. A., and Royal, C. (eds.). *Lessons from the Field: Applying Appreciative Inquiry.* Plano, Tex.: Thin Book, 1998.

Hart, E. "Executive Leadership Teams: Exorcising Demons, Exercising Minds." *Planning Review,* 1995, *23*(4), 14–19, 46.

Hawley, J. *Reawakening the Spirit in Work: The Power of Dharmic Management.* San Francisco: Berrett-Koehler, 1993.

Helgesen, S. *The Female Advantage: Women's Ways of Leadership.* New York: Doubleday Currency, 1990.

Hersey, P. *Situational Leadership: A Summary.* Escondido, Calif.: Center for Leadership Studies, 1993.

Holpp, L., and Phillips, R. "When Is a Team Its Own Worst Enemy?" *Training,* 1995, *32*(9), 71–82.

Horak, B. J. "Building a Team on a Medical Floor." *Health Care Management Review,* 1991, *16*(2), 65–71.

Hout, T. M., and Carter, J. C. "Getting It Done: New Roles for Senior Executives." *Harvard Business Review,* 1995 (Nov./Dec.), 133–145.

Huret, J. "Paying for Team Results." *HR Magazine,* 1991 (May), 39–41.

Jacobsen-Webb, M. "Team Building: Key to Executive Success." *Journal of Nursing Administration*, 1985, *15*(2), 16–20.

Kim, W. C., and Mauborgne, R. A. "Parables of Leadership." *Harvard Business Review*, 1992 (July/Aug.), 123–128.

Kohles, M. K., Baker, W. G., and Donaho, B. A. *Transformational Leadership: Renewing Fundamental Values and Achieving New Relationships in Health Care.* Chicago: American Hospital Association, 1995.

Leander, W. "Layered Learning: Improved Learning Through Phased Education." *Patient Focused Care Association Review*, 1994 (summer), 2–7.

Linden, R. M. "Flattening the Hierarchy Through Self-Managing Teams: I." *Virginia Review*, 1992a (Oct.), 52–53.

Linden, R. M. "Self-Managing Teams II: Dealing with the Issues." *Virginia Review*, 1992b (Nov.), 20–21.

Lumsdon, K. "Why Executive Teams Fail and What to Do." *Hospitals & Health Networks*, Aug. 5, 1995, pp. 24–31.

Manion, J. "Chaos or Transformation? Managing the Process of Innovation." In S. S. Blanchett and D. L. Flarey (eds.), *Process-Centered Health Care Organizations.* Gaithersburg, Md.: Aspen, 1999.

Manthey, M. "An Expert Answers Common Questions About Primary Nursing." *Nursing Management*, 1989, *20*(3), 22–24.

Manthey, M., and Miller, D. "Tools for Leaders, Tools for Managers." *Nursing Management*, 1991, *22*(11), 20–21.

McNeese-Smith, D. "The Impact of Leadership on Productivity." *Nursing Economics*, 1992, *10*(6), 393–396.

McNeese-Smith, D. "Leadership Behavior and Employee Effectiveness." *Nursing Management*, 1993, *24*(5), 38–39.

McNeese-Smith, D. "A Nursing Shortage: Building Organizational Commitment Among Nurses." *Journal of Healthcare Management*, 2001, *46*(3), 173–187.

Moffitt, G., McCullough, C., and Sanders, D. "High-Performing Self-Directed Work Teams: What Are They and How Do They Work?" *Patient Focused Care Association Review*, 1993 (fall), 8–12.

Moss-Kanter, R. *When Giants Learn to Dance: Mastering the Challenge of Strategy, Management and Career in the 1990s.* New York: Simon & Schuster, 1989.

Naisbett, J. *Megatrends: Ten New Directions Transforming Our Lives.* New York: Warner Books, 1982.

Naisbett, J., and Aburdene, P. *Megatrends 2000: Ten New Directions for the 1990s.* New York: Morrow, 1990.

O'Dell, C. "Team Play, Team Pay: New Ways of Keeping Score." *Across the Board*, 1989 (Nov.), 31–45.

Orsburn, J. D., Moran, L., Musselwhite, E., and Zenger, J. *Self-Directed Work Teams: The New American Challenge*. Homewood, Ill.: Business One Irwin, 1990.

Peters, T., and Waterman, R. *In Search of Excellence: Lessons from America's Best-Run Companies*. New York: HarperCollins, 1982.

Ranney, J., and Deck, M. "Making Teams Work: Lessons from the Leaders in New Product Development." *Planning Review*, 1995, *23*(4), 6–13.

Reddy, W. B. *Intervention Skills: Process Consultation for Small Groups and Teams*. San Diego: Pfeiffer, 1994.

Saarel, D. "Triads: Self-Organizing Structures That Create Value." *Planning Review*, 1995, *23*(4), 20–25.

Schrubb, D. A. "The Implementation of Self-Managed Teams in Health Care." *Topics in Health Information Management*, 1992, *13*(1), 45–50.

Schwarz, R. "Becoming a Facilitative Leader." *Training and Development*, 2003 (Apr.), 51–57.

Scott, C. D., and Jaffe, D. T. *Managing Organizational Change*. Menlo Park, Calif.: Crisp, 1989a.

Scott, C. D., and Jaffe, D. T. *Managing Personal Change*. Menlo Park, Calif.: Crisp, 1989b.

Scott, C. D., and Jaffe, D. T. "From Crisis to Culture Change." *Healthcare Forum Journal*, 1991, *34*(3), 31–39.

Scott, C. D., Jaffe, D. T., and Tobe, M. *Organizational Vision, Values and Mission*. Menlo Park, Calif.: Crisp, 1993.

Shelton, C. "Team Mania." *Executive Excellence*, 1995 (June), 9–10.

Sherer, J. "Tapping into Teams." *Hospitals & Health Networks*, July 5, 1995, pp. 32–36.

Siebert, A. *The Survivor Personality*. Portland, Oreg.: Practical Psychology Press, 1993.

Smith, S. P., and Flarey, D. L. (eds.). *Process-Centered Health Care Organizations*. Gaithersburg, Md.: Aspen, 1999.

Spencer, S. A., and Adams, J. D. *Life Changes: Growing Through Personal Transitions*. San Luis Obispo, Calif.: Impact, 1990.

Tjosvold, D., and Tjosvold, M. *Leading the Team Organization: How to Create an Enduring Competitive Advantage*. New York: Lexington Books, 1991.

Tuckman, B. W. "Developmental Sequence in Small Groups." *Psychological Bulletin*, 1965, *63*(6), 334–399.

Voluntary Hospitals of America. *Improving Patient Outcomes Through System Change: A Focus on Changing Roles of Health Care Organization Executives.* Irving, Tex.: Voluntary Hospitals of America, 1994.

Warner, M. "Why Teams Fail, How Teams Succeed." *Executive Excellence,* 1995 (June), 17.

Wellins, R., Byham, W., and Wilson, J. *Empowered Teams: Creating Self-Directed Work Groups That Improve Quality, Productivity, and Participation.* San Francisco: Jossey-Bass, 1991.

Wellins, R., and George, J. "The Key to Self-Directed Work Teams." *Training,* 1991 (Apr.), 26–31.

Wilson, J., and Wellins, R. "Leading Teams." *Executive Excellence,* 1995 (June), 7–8.

Yager, E. "Coaching Teams." *Executive Excellence,* 1995 (June), 8.

Zemke, R. "Rethinking the Rush to Team Up." *Training,* 1993, 30(11), 55–61.

Zenger, J., Musselwhite, E., Hurson, K., and Perrin, C. *Leading Teams: Mastering the New Role.* Homewood, Ill.: Business One Irwin, 1994.

Index